The Baby Boomers Beauty Bible

The natural way to beautiful skin at any age

By

Jan Benham

Author of
The Creamy Craft of Cosmetic Making
With essential oils and their friends
& The Little Book of lipsticks

Published in 2011 by Antony Rowe
Publishing
48-50 Birch Close
Eastbourne
East Sussex
BN23 6PE
arp@cpi-group.co.uk

© Jan Benham 2011

A catalogue record for this book is available
from the British Library

ISBN 978-1-907571-21-3

Printed and Bound in Great Britain by
CPI Antony Rowe, Chippenham and
Eastbourne

Acknowledgements

I thank my family and friends who have supported me in getting this book finished and to press. I am deeply gratefully to my loving mother, Jacqui Benham who showed me how to connect to my intuition, and my father, Ken Benham, who believed in me and told me that my dreams can become my realities. I would also like to thank my wonderful son, Glyn Morgan, who is such a big help with my public relations and in teaching at the school.

A big hug and a thank you to my current staff and teachers at the Institute: Tomoko Yamaji, Eri Nose, Rani M. Johnson, Violet A. Cordy, Danielle Murray, and Doctor Helena Ovens.

To Ian Brealey at Shirley price Aromatherapy, UK and all the staff.

Thank you my beautiful students and loyal clients for inspiring me to experiment, create and continue to grow.

Lowess, my dearest friend, you are the inspiration for 'Inner Care.'

To Jan kloosterhuis with love

Table of Contents

Foreword

I have often commented to myself at Jan Benham's glowing complexion and youthful appearance, for a number of years now. As a doctor of Naturopathy, I focus my attention on the prevention and treatment of disease. It often manifests as a combination of emotional/mental, physical and spiritual imbalances.

After reading this book, I have nothing but praise for her holistic approach to skin care. I agree wholeheartedly with her emphasis on the importance that the skin plays in the health and well-being of the individual. The skin is the largest organ system of the body which both absorbs nutrients and eliminates waste materials.

In this toxic world, we need to be aware of the importance of substances that we put on our skin. Forty years of sun block, for instance, has likely contributed to the epidemic of osteoporosis that we see today by preventing the conversion of sunlight to Vitamin D.

Jan has given us a multitude of viable (and wonderful) alternatives to the chemically-laden products that are currently on the market. Most people are now aware of the harmful effects of the pesticides and preservatives that are in our food. Trends have changed to a preference for organic foods which are as healthy for our external environment as they are for our internal environment. Until now, the same could not be said for our cosmetics industry.

Here is a book that offers consumers the opportunity to take another important step towards manifesting a healthy lifestyle by choosing to use natural non-toxic creams and lotions.

I wish Jan the very best success in the launch of her second edition of her book.

Helena Ovens, N.D., FCAH, CCH, CBHT

Preface to the Second edition

This second edition....

Just as my first book *The Creamy Craft of Cosmetic Making; with Essential Oils and their Friends,* arose in response to the many requests by therapists in the healing profession, this book concentrates on natural approaches to combating ageing. This second edition adds new content, expands on previous coverage, and addresses important new themes to enhance the experience of using aromatherapy. The changing climate of the beauty field, and heightened awareness of the types of harmful substances that may appear in beauty products, has meant there is more desire for information regarding natural products. Therefore, in this edition I have tried to provide information for therapists and interested home producers, with more explanation and more explicit instruction.

Back in 1995, unscented lotions and creams were available from chemists (or drugstores if you're in Canada or the US), for custom blending but they were full of chemicals and petroleum by-products. Instead therapists, including myself, wanted more control over what went into their products. In particular, Aromatherapists wanted to custom blend their own creams and lotions. So *voila!* This book and the *Creamy Craft of Cosmetic Making* were born.

While I expected people to enjoy making their own lotions and creams, as I enjoy it so much, I have been overwhelmed by the high interest. I have constantly been asked (on a daily basis), when a new version of my book would be out.

Since 1995, after hundreds of classes teaching the cream-making course to therapists from all over the world, and also since the first edition of this book was published, much more information has come to light about the various emulsifiers that can be used for cream making. After looking at the food industry, I discovered other emulsifiers that make fabulous creams and give the cream maker a choice of products and a chance to make something a little different.

The development of home-made commercial grade shampoos and conditioners became a course in its own right. As a result, this book includes information and recipes for making your very own hair shampoos, conditioners and hair treatments plus body washes.

Though *The Baby Boomers Beauty Bible* is best read as a sequel to *The Creamy Craft of Cosmetic Making*, it includes enough of the basics to be read as a stand-alone work.

Happy beauty product making!

PART ONE

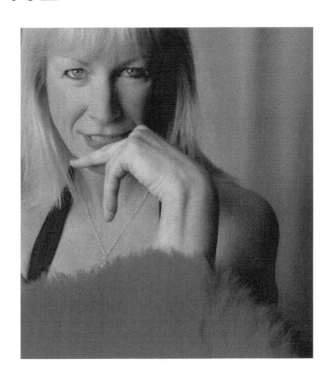

Introduction to Skin Care

The skin is our body's largest organ. As well as acting as a protective barrier for our body, it breathes, detoxifies, and regulates our body temperature.

Everything about our body and mind seems to show up in our skin, especially, on the face. Have you noticed that every time you have a hot date, a big zit magically appears on your nose?

Our skin is like a mirror to our inner self. How we take care of ourselves physically, emotionally, spiritually, mentally and sexually shows up in some form or other on our skin.

If we change just one aspect of our life, whether it be how we take care of ourselves physically, or emotionally, for example, it will have impact on all the other aspects. True beauty lies within – when we feel good, we look good, and when we look good, we feel good.

Caring for ourselves with natural, time-honoured products, both internally and externally, brings its rewards too. Your skin is your connection between yourself and the outside world and, therefore, greatly reflects how you relate to the world and how the world sees you. By nurturing skin and giving it what it needs, you can achieve skin that accurately reflects your inner beauty. Your skin is your body's "protective coating," and so taking steps to influence the health of your skin is important.

So my aim is to give you a guideline, a discipline to follow. If you work on your skin, hair and body on a daily basis for three months, I guarantee change will occur on many levels. You will start to feel good about yourself and self empowered. Your relationships with yourself and significant others will shift, so be warned.

Consider a more natural route to a vibrant complexion though skincare that uses simple plant-based ingredients.

Skin Care – A Quick Anatomy Lesson

The skin is composed of 70% water, 27% protides, 2% lipids, and 1% lucides and has two layers – the **epidermis** and the **dermis.** The epidermis is the outermost layer and acts as a physical barrier, protecting the underlying organs. The inner dermis contains numerous blood vessels, protein fibres, sweat glands and sebaceous glands.

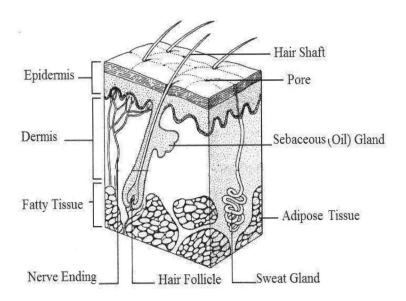

General Skin Functions

The skin has the ability to:

- Protect against wounds and micro-organisms. The skin is in continuous contact with micro-organisms. Skin is acidic (pH of 5.5 to 6.2); it effectively blocks micro-organisms from entering. It is important that we maintain the skin's pH balance as it helps the body's defence system.

- Protect against the sun or natural radiation. Keratin and melanin rise from the basal cell layer of the epidermis toward the upper layers and tan to prevent burning. Sebum and sweat (including your stored leukocytes) also defend the body against ultra violet rays.

- Act as a waterproof barrier – Water does not penetrate because of the horny cells – formed from dead skin cells, keratin, fatty tissues and sebum.

- Withstand physical influences. It is able to absorb external shock and pressures.

- Breathe oxygen – The skin tissues breathe. Oxygen is absorbed and carbon dioxide is exhaled.

- Regulate the temperature of the body – sweat glands produce perspiration. The evaporation of perspiration from the skin's surface cools the body, thus maintaining the body's temperature.

- Secrete wastes – Perspiration contains a small percentage of waste which helps rid the body of toxins. Sweat glands are most numerous on the palms of the hands and the soles of the feet. Sweat glands react to adrenaline stimulation which is why some people suffer from sweaty hands when they are nervous or anxious. Sebaceous glands produce sebum, the body's natural oil which also forces out harmful substances. Sebaceous glands are most numerous on the face, scalp, upper back and chest.

- Feel sensations – The skin contains nerve endings which make us aware of our surroundings. They act as a warning system to indicate heat, cold, pain, pressure and other external factors.

- Absorb substances – The skin can absorb certain vitamins, essential oils, herbal extracts, chemicals and hormones.

- Synthesize – The skin aids in the production of vitamin D from sunlight.

- Regenerate – Beauty and freshness of the skin depends on the speed with which the skin can regenerate itself – usually 30-90 days depending on age.

So let's get started by following the next few pages to a more youthful and vibrant you.

Choosing Ingredients

Some cream makers make products just for themselves while others are trying to supplement or even supplant family incomes. The idea that what we put into our body affects our health has now become accepted and, it is now known that certain chemicals and hormones are absorbed through the skin. The use of oestrogen patches is just one example of how the medical profession is utilizing this knowledge. Because of this understanding, there has been a huge growth in the natural cream and cosmetic making industry.

Benefits of Home Production

Individuals are uniquely positioned to make better beauty products than companies that do mass production. Small producers work on a smaller scale, have more control over the production process, and can make choices that a large producer is restricted from. Independent producers who value locally produced materials, or natural or organic products have control over, and can make decisions about, their own ingredient choices, and by extension, what they consume through their skin. Personal control over production allows small producers like yourself, to monitor what goes into the products and the standards of cleanliness they use. Also, as an independent producer, you maintain control over your own safety and work standards of production. This ensures that you are using cosmetics made by workers who are treated fairly rather than supporting companies who may take advantage of their workers.

Large producers often find it necessary to turn to non-natural alternatives. Due to difficulties finding enough high-quality natural products, or sources that can maintain a steady supply, they turn to cheaper and easier methods of production. Synthetic ingredients are accessible, stable and economical, so they are often used to replace natural ones. Even when manufacturers do incorporate organic nutrients, the percentages are rather insignificant – eye-catching on the label and inconspicuous in the product.

Consumers often have little or no understanding of products' ingredients and many people have allergic reactions to one item or the other, usually due to the use of petroleum-based material, or other synthetic materials, fragrance, colourants, or preservatives.

To quote from *The Cure For All Diseases* by Hulda Regehr Clark, Ph.D., ND:

> People are trying desperately to use less toxic products. They seek health for themselves. So they reach for products that just list herbs and other natural ingredients. Unfortunately, the buyers are being duped. The Food and Drug Administration (FDA) requires all body products to have sufficient antiseptic in them. Some of these antiseptics are substances you must avoid! But you won't see them on a label because manufacturers prefer to use quantities below the levels they must disclose. (1993, p. 436)

Some of the unnatural chemicals listed are present because of residues in the manufacturing process, like Propyl alcohol and wood alcohol, which are present because the tubing used to fill the bottles is sterilized and cleaned using them.

Benzene can be found in toothpaste while hair spray contains propyl alcohol and PCBs. Shampoos and creams all contain sulphates and propyl glycol (that's anti-freeze!), to name just a few of the dangerous chemicals present.

So the crafty home cosmetic maker can have so much more control and meet family skin-care needs better than industry can.

Know Your Ingredients

For further awareness of chemicals to avoid, and also information about the ingredients mentioned in this book please read on.

First of all understand that everything can be broken down into chemical components. So when I mention alcohol, it doesn't mean an alcoholic beverage. All essential oils for example, are naturally made up of a composite of chemicals including esters, alcohols, aldehydes, ketones, phenols, oxides and terpenes.

There are chemicals that are helpful to us and chemicals that are downright dangerous. Below is a discussion of just a few of the worst offenders.

Chemicals that Harm

Benzene

Benzene is known to be a carcinogen. Harmful amounts may be absorbed through the skin; it is irritating to the mucous membranes and poisonous when ingested. Because it is usually a trace element, it will not show up on the list of ingredients of cosmetics.

Colours and dyes (FD & C, or D & C)

Artificial colours are made from petroleum and coal tar, and are believed to be cancer causing agents. They penetrate the skin, can cause allergies and are irritants to the skin and eyes. They are found on labels as FD&C, or D&C and are followed by a colour and a number.

DEA (diethanolamine)

This is a synthetic solvent, detergent and humectants widely used in brake fluid, industrial degreasers and antifreeze. It is mostly used in liquid soap, shampoo and conditioner. It can be harmful for the liver, kidneys and pancreas. It may cause cancer in various organs. Irritates skin, eyes, and mucous membranes and is a health risk especially to infants and young children.

Formaldehyde

Due to its bad reputation, it is sometimes hidden under the name DMDM hydantoin or MDM hydantoin. The trade name is Formalin. A common ingredient in shampoos, it is a disinfectant, germicide and fungicide and is used as a preservative in shampoos. There is a suspected link to some cancers and it also causes a breakdown of DNA in the skin. Unfortunately, due to the fact that formaldehyde is often used as a preservative in surfactants (washing substance), it is not often listed as an ingredient.

Parabens (methyl, ethyl, propyl and benzyl)

Cheap preservatives used in beauty-care products that make it possible for them to survive the long trip from China, sit on store or warehouse shelves for years or be exposed to extreme temperatures. When parabens are applied as a cream, the chemicals appear in the blood within hours. Parabens have been shown to mimic oestrogen, disrupting our bodies' endocrine (hormone) system and have been found in human breast tumours possibly linking them to breast cancer. Where possible use glass containers for your personal beauty products.

Propyl Alcohol (also known as isopropyl alcohol and rubbing alcohol)

Unfortunately propyl alcohol is not on the list of ingredients as it is used as an antiseptic in the bottling procedure, so theoretically it is not an ingredient. Traces can be found though in most cosmetics, creams, shampoos etc. Possible effects of propyl alcohol include mental depression, headaches and even cancer. The fatal ingested dose is 1 fluid ounce.

Phthalates

Phthalates are industrial chemicals that

make plastics soft. They are found in over 70 percent of beauty products and are absorbed through the skin. They have been found to cause birth defects, infertility and other illnesses. If you use plastics, try to transfer the contents to glass containers when possible.

Propylene Glycol (common name Antifreeze)

Propylene glycol is the main ingredient in anti-freeze, brake and hydraulic fluid. I personally know of one person whose beloved dog died by ingesting antifreeze. Propylene glycol, the most widely used cosmetic ingredient is found in moisturisers, baby lotions, makeup, shampoos and hair conditioners. Material safety data sheets on propylene glycol warn users to avoid skin contact as it is systemic and can cause liver abnormalities and kidney damage. Note: it is widely used in baby wipes.

Sodium Lauryl Sulphate and Sodium Laureth Sulphate

Up to 50% of most shampoos are made up of these ingredients. Originally invented to clean garage floors, SLS has been linked to cataracts and cancer. SLS can actually damage the outer layer of the skin, causing dryness, scaliness, and loss of flexibility. SLS denatures protein and can change genetic material found in cells (mutagenic).

Synthetic Perfumes

Fragrance is used extensively in skin and hair care products and is often the leading cause if allergies and skin

Alkyl-phenol ethoxylades

problems. Complaints to the FDA concerning perfumes include headaches, dizziness, violent coughing, vomiting and skin irritations and rashes.

This ingredient is used in the production of shampoo making. Its chemicals mimic oestrogen causing havoc with lowered sperm counts. It has also been linked to breast cancer from the high levels of oestrogen.

I could write a whole book about dangerous chemicals, but this gives you some idea about what people are using in the commercial market place for beauty products.

Let's turn now to the ingredients that can contribute to good health and glowing skin.

Chemicals that Heal

Algae powder (Laminaria digitata and Fucus vesiculosus)

These are powerful detoxifiers and absorb toxins on the skin without harming the living skin. At the Aromashoppe, we use algae which has been freeze dried. It becomes active again when it is put into water. We use it in body wraps and as a bath blend. It detoxifies not only the skin, but the whole body, making it a wonderful treatment for cellulite and fluid retention.

Carrier oils

A carrier oil is a vegetable oil derived from plants, (from the seeds, kernels or nuts). Each carrier oil differs in the therapeutic properties and characteristics that they offer. For example, sesame oil has a sun protection factor of four. While sesame, jojoba, almond, or apricot kernel oils are true carrier oils, *infused* oils such as calendula and carrot root (used in many of the recipes in this book) are infused with herbs and roots within a base carrier oil and therefore have additional therapeutic benefits. In choosing carrier oils for use in natural beauty products, choose cold-pressed versions where possible.

Coco palm emulsifying wax
(Chemical name: Cetyl stearyl alcohol)

This emulsifying wax is derived naturally from the fatty acids of palm and coconut oils.

Conditioning emulsifier

This is a blend of cetearyl alcohol, castor oil, and stearalkonium chloride. This emulsifying wax improves the ability to detangle the hair and adds shine.

Cornacopa
(Chemical name: Decyl polyglucose)

This is made from re-growable raw materials – glucose derived from corn and fatty alcohols from coconut and palm kernel oils. Although cornacopa has been around for years, the use was previously limited by the lack of a large scale commercial plant. Cornacopa is biodegradable, earth-friendly, orally non-toxic and very mild to the skin and eyes. It can make up to 50% of the shampoo.

Essential oils

Essential oils are extracted by various methods, usually steam distillation from plants, herbs, flowers, trees, seeds and grasses. They have been used in skin and health care for thousands of years and have marvellous therapeutic capabilities. For example, Lavender's delightful and soothing scent also provides antiseptic and analgesic effects. For further reading, the *Creamy Craft of Cosmetic Making* has a whole chapter devoted to this subject.

Grapefruit seed extract

A by-product of the citrus industry, grapefruit seed extract contains vitamin C and glycerin. Grapefruit seed extract is anti-bacterial, anti-microbial, antiseptic, and can be used internally to combat fungus infections. As a result, this makes a natural preservative for creams, lotions and cosmetics, etc.

Lanette wax

Did you know that there are 600 lanette waxes on the market and most that are sold contain sodium laurel sulphate (see *Chemicals that Harm*). The one sold at my Aromashoppe contains just cetyl stearyl alcohol, a safe chemical naturally derived from the fatty acids of coconut oil.

Seaweed extract and gel (red algae)

Seaweed is an anti-oxidant and is full of easy to absorb proteins, vitamins, minerals and lipids. Repairing and protecting the skin and hair, it reduces oiliness and sebum over-production and strengthens against damage caused by free radicals.

Wheat protein

This adds protection for the skin and hair as it moisturises and softens. Wheat

19

protein strengthens the elasticity of the hair and repairs damage to the hair especially hair that has been overly processed and coloured. When added to the shampoo, the wheat protein can make the shampoo into an all-in-one shampoo and conditioner.

Xanthan gum A gum produced by a pure culture fermentation of a carbohydrate with *xanthomonas campestris*, this is widely used as a thickener in the cosmetic and food industries.

The Power of Botanicals

We have been primping, perfuming, and decorating our bodies since the beginning of time to enhance our attractiveness and magnetism. While we've given up practices like face masks made of crocodile manure and lead paint for whitening the skin, natural skincare has always had an enduring attraction. Since Cleopatra's time, botanical extracts have remained the most important resource for healing and beautifying in the natural world.

Since flowers first appeared on the earth, humans have been fascinated by them. These beautiful and aromatic plants were the first to be valued only for their gift, without seeming to have a purpose. Botanicals simply exist to be enjoyed and to be appreciated for their beauty.

Flowers have provided inspiration and pleasure for centuries. Whether you are an artist, a poet, or simply someone who enjoys nature, seeing the beauty in a flower or in its scent, links us all to the secrets of the universe. The first time someone recognized the beauty of flowers and of their scents, was a major step toward our human awakened consciousness. This contact with the sentiments of delight, pleasure, appreciation, and gratitude, set us on the path to enlightenment. They opened us to universal connection, compassion, and loving kindness. Flowers have even inspired mystics. As Eckhart Tolle discusses:

> Jesus tells us to contemplate the flowers and learn from them how to live. The Buddha is said to have given a 'silent sermon' once during which he held up a flower and gazed at it. After a while, one of those present, a monk called Mahakasyapa, began to smile. He is said to have been the only one who had understood the sermon. According to legend, that smile (that is to say, realization) was handed down by twenty-eight successive masters and much later became the origin of Zen. (2006, p. 2-3)

As flowers are vulnerable, delicate and last only for a short time, they embody a message to make contact with the ephemeral, the sacred, and the spiritual within ourselves. Flowers and floral essences can help awaken us to our inner beauty. They are like a bridge to the world of the ethereal and remind us to stay in contact with a world beyond our everyday reality.

The selection of botanical extracts is both an art and a science. The fragrance contributes to both our psychological and physiological well being. There is a long history of remedies associated with most botanicals.

Each botanical makes its own unique contribution to your healing, however used in combination; the synergy goes beyond what each delivers on its own. This is why you will often see distinctive blends that provide a combination of important botanicals in creams, lotions and ointments.

Important Considerations in Natural Cosmetic Making

Remember that not all ingredients are equal. Just because they have the same name, they are not necessarily the same quality. For example, there are many types of lanette wax, along with differing quality levels. Be cautious about your choice of products, as they will be used on your face and body. To be confident, buy only from reputable organizations that you know and trust.

Be especially vigilant when purchasing essential oils as some less-reputable producers will dilute, or tamper with essential oils that are difficult or expensive to produce. Essential oils including Rose, Melissa, Jasmine or Neroli, are often targeted by adding alcohol, synthetic products, or other cheaper oils, such as in the case of Neroli, Petitgrain is often added to *stretch* the more expensive oil. The addition of cheaper oils or synthetic products can radically change or reduce the therapeutic properties and the healing value of the oil. Also, unpleasant side effects such as skin irritations and nausea may occur. A true essential oil is extracted from herbs, grasses, seeds, fruits, flowers, leaves, roots, or bark. Extraction from some plants is a long and difficult process, resulting in high investments of both time and money, and consequently selling prices can be quite high. This is one reason why artificial products are so often used in the mass market. Therefore, if the price of an essential oil seems too good to be true, it probably is.

In some stores, even natural products may have been sitting on the shelf for a year or more, so as a consumer you need to be attentive. In making your own products, you have more control over their quality.

As a producer you must be aware of the date you produced your products, as they will eventually expire. Rancidity happens when vegetable-based oils oxidize and start to smell bad. Some creams made with hemp seed oil will turn rancid within 6 months while others that are made with jojoba oil will never go rancid because jojoba is technically a liquid wax. However, some skin creams are already damaged by free radicals even before the product goes rancid. To protect yourself and your family, use only fresh products that you know have been made within the last six months.

Note that when you use dairy products like cream or yogurt, just as you would not eat something that was stale, expired or that had gone bad (or that simply had not been kept in the refrigerator), you need to take the same extra care with your ski
When making your own products, to prevent the transmission of infection, be sure to wash your hands properly, paying attention to your nails and cuticles. It is important to **use sterile gloves and a hair net** to provide necessary protection.

Proper Measurement

Ounces	Drams	Spoons	cc's	ml's
1/8	=1	=1/2 tsp.	= 2	= 2
1/4	=2	=1 tsp.	= 5	= 5
1/3	=3	=1 dsp.[1]	= 10	= 10
1/2	=4	=1 tbsp.	= 15	= 15
1	=8	=2 tbsp.	=30	= 30
4	=32	=4 tbsp.	=120	=120

Note: In the recipes you will often see reference to a *dollop*. A dollop is large drop or a squeeze. For example, you will note that a dollop is mentioned when adding Carrot root oil, Vitamin E, Grapefruit seed extract or Benzoin resinoid to the creams, shampoos and lotion.

Note. When measuring either the lanette wax or cocopalm emulsifying wax, 4 heaped dsp. makes 1 oz. weight.

Now, let's make the basics.

---

[1] dsp. = dessert spoon (this spoon is a size between a teaspoon and a tablespoon, a 10 ml spoon)

The Essential Guide to
Basic Cream and Lotion Making

Tools of the Trade

It is always important to have the proper equipment. Fortunately, cream and shampoo making uses basic kitchenware.

So to begin, you will need the following equipment:

- A double boiler (or a pot and a heat resistant glass bowl you can place over the pot filled with boiling water)

- A stainless steel saucepan.

- A measuring jug – one litre size preferred.

- A wooden spoon.

- Measuring spoons
  (i.e., teaspoon (5 ml), dessertspoon (10 ml), and tablespoon (15 ml))

- A scale that will measure ounces and metrics (available at most kitchen suppliers).

- Empty jars and bottles for creams, toners and shampoos, etc. *(I prefer glass ones).*

- Labels (so you can keep your final products organized).

- A hand held blender.

- Moulds for making bath bombs.

Each time you use it, clean all equipment in boiling water, rinse well and dry. It is best to use these utensils only for making cosmetics and not to prepare or store food in them due to the possibility of cross-contamination.

Cautions

- Pay attention when heating any mixtures that include oil! It can rapidly overheat!

- If the phone or doorbell goes, remove pan from heat. Small amounts of oils can overheat in seconds if left unattended.

- Do not overheat the oils. The wax and oil mixtures merely need to be melted, not boiled to death.

- Keep a bottle of Lavender nearby in case you are burnt by oil.

- Keep young children and pets out of the way.

- Immediately remove any oil or cream that has spilled on the floor.

Basic Instructions

Lotion and Cream Making

1. Sterilize all utensils, product containers, and workshop surfaces. Wipe utensils and wipe down surfaces with alcohol.

2. In a heat resistant bowl (or in a double boiler), melt the emulsifying waxes, butters and oils.

3. In another saucepan, heat the liquid ingredients (hydrosols (Rose water, etc.), Witch Hazel, distilled water, etc.) until they have reached boiling point.

4. When the waxes and oils have completely melted, and the water is gently boiling…

5. Slowly, add the waters to the melted waxes and oils, stirring constantly, until all water has been added.

6. Remove the double boiler from the heat source. Continue stirring until the mixture has completely cooled.

7. Add natural preservative, plus any essential oils, nutrients and goodies.

8. Pour into sterilized jars and bottles.

9. Label.

Try out some trial batches first until you get the hang of cream making. This will avoid waste and also allow for experimentation. Quite often, I have found that the less likely combinations become favourites.

So let's get started!

Experimental Basic Lotion

This trial-sized batch makes one 120 ml (4oz) bottle of lotion.

INGREDIENTS:

Waxes:
  1 tsp. (5ml) Lanette wax or cocopalm emulsifying wax
  1 tbsp. (15ml) Fractionated Coconut oil
Waters:
  50 ml Rose water
  100 ml Distilled water
  1 drop Myrrh
Optional:
  1 dollop Grapefruit seed extract

METHOD:

Follow the *Basic Instructions* (see page 29).

Experimental Basic Cream

This trial-sized batch makes one 60ml (2oz) jar of cream.

INGREDIENTS:

Waxes and oils:
> **1 tsp. (5 ml)** Lanette wax or cocopalm emulsifying wax
> **1 tbsp. (15 ml)** Fractionated Coconut oil

Waters:
> **20 ml** Rose water
> **50 ml** Distilled water
> **1 drop** Myrrh

Optional:
> **1 dollop** Grapefruit seed extract

METHOD:
Follow the *Basic Instructions*.

Note: the difference between lotion and cream is the amount of water in the recipe.

PART
FOUR

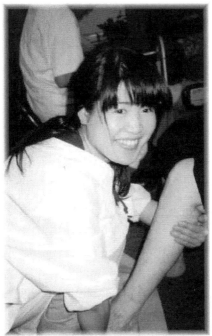

Photo: Jan Benham

Inner Care

*It is important to treat our skin from both angles:
inner and outer.*

At the Institute, we study the care of the skin from both the inside and the outside.

The results are amazing. Often students with some form of skin problem at the beginning of their course, begin to show signs of skin improvement by the time they complete their training.

Following these tips will result not only in beautiful, radiant skin but will also decrease the risk of encountering many major diseases that can shorten peoples' lives or compromise their quality of life considerably.

Water the rose from the root

Reduce Toxins

To achieve inner balance, know what to remove from your life. While this could be a book in itself, briefly here are some suggestions.

Remove as many toxins as you can from your environment (plastic water bottles, plastic wrap in the microwave or harsh household cleaners) and get educated about the environment. There are many books available on this topic and you will find some of them recommended in the 'Further Reading' section of this book.

A major contributor to our health is what we put in our mouths.

Top 10 list of foods and drinks to avoid

1. Refined sugar, fizzy drinks or pop.

2. Fast food such as pizza, burgers and fries

3. Hydrogenated - or trans-fats (ingredients used in biscuits, crackers or cookies) and olestra (a synthetic fat that is banned in some places).

4. Excessive caffeine (over one cup of coffee a day).

5. Chemical food additives and Nitrates (used for curing bacon, hot dogs and other processed meats)

6. Alcohol (except for moderate amounts of red wine)

7. Products made with refined white flour.

8. Saturated animal fats (Consumption of over 4 ounces of protein every day is ill-advised).

9. High-fat foods (including, snacks, chips, cookies, and the majority of processed foods).

10. High-sodium foods.

Additional non-food triggers of ageing skin include:

- Over exposure to UVA rays – destroys elastin and collagen fibres

- Skin creams already damaged by free radicals (note that this can occur before the product goes rancid.)

- Air pollution

- Prolonged emotional stress

- Insufficient nutrition

- Exposure to sulphates and chemicals that are in our skin, body and hair care products

- Tobacco

Follow proper nutrition

The more pretty colours you eat, the lovelier you will be.
Healthy is as healthy eats, so here's the rainbow for thee!

Hydrate

The most important thing to do for your skin is to drink enough water. Suggested amounts are two litres per day.

Eat your veggies.

Although many different treatments and products can assist in improving the look of your skin, the first step is to feed it and protect it through a healthy lifestyle,

You should eat at least 5 servings of fruits and vegetables a day.

Maintain Fats and Proteins

I have found that a big cause of ageing is too little fat and protein in our diets. I see some people (mostly women) who by the time they are 35 years old, already look old beyond their years, because they cut all fats from their diets and don't eat enough protein (which affects the collagen and elastin fibres in our skin).

Incorporate Antioxidants

"Antioxidants", the new buzz word, are described as health powerhouses and key nutrients to our health. We need to seek balance between so-called "good" nutrients (like antioxidants) and "bad" (like free radicals - some call these "cell-killers"). When our balance is off, we age faster and move toward disease faster.

What are "free radicals"?
Sometimes the body creates a chemical reaction that breaks the bonds that hold paired electrons together inside a cell, and free radicals are produced. These unpaired or "rogue" electrons try to steal partners for them from other molecules. These attacks damage the body's cells - a process called oxidation (similar to when fruits turn brown, a nail rusts, or butter turns rancid). While our bodies produce free radicals naturally, when produced in excess they can damage the cells (the membranes, genetic material in cells (DNA), fatty acids and other body structures). Also, they commence a chain reaction which perpetuates the problem.

Studies show that free radicals increase:
- Our rate of ageing
- The prevalence of cancer (by damaging the body's cells).
- Damage to the lens of the eye (and may lead to blindness).
- Inflammation and joint problems, such as arthritis.
- Autoimmune diseases (like Crohn's disease, endometriosis, fibromyalgia, diabetes and lupus).

- Cardiovascular disease (like high blood pressure, stroke, or heart attack) (by increasing the incidence of LDL ("bad") cholesterol)

- Brain cell damage (promoting neurological conditions such as Parkinson's or Alzheimer's disease)

- The prevalence of cancer (by damaging the body's cells).

What are Antioxidants?

Antioxidant molecules defend the body by ending the chain reaction started by free radicals before vital molecules can be damaged. Although our bodies have a natural ability to produce antioxidants, overwork may tax the body's normal antioxidant production system and leave it unable to cope. We need to pay more attention to antioxidants in our diet these days to counteract our unhealthy lifestyle, its high stress level, and the increasing number of toxins we encounter in our environment. The most commonly-known antioxidants are vitamins A, C and E (the 'ACE' vitamins); and the minerals selenium, copper and zinc. Recently, many other naturally occurring anti-oxidants have been discovered in plants.

Choosing Antioxidants

One important trick to incorporating antioxidants into your diet is to choose foods from different colour palettes. Just as Mother Nature's garden blooms with all the colours of the rainbow, the spectrum of purples, blues, greens, yellows, oranges and reds carries her bounty as well. The beauty and vitality in these colours gives us important hints about the built-in nutrition and healing powers of common foods and herbs. Antioxidant boosters tend to have the deepest, darkest colours, like jewels. This is because the sun works to infuse the plants with all the colours of the rainbow. By rewarding our senses, the colours of vitality provide clues about the properties of healing foods. So choose a "colour wheel" of varied colours to be sure you gain as much benefit as you can from the food you eat. Try to vary from colours you have eaten earlier in the day, or the week.

Add supplements

Herbal extracts whether drunk as a tea or taken internally as a tincture, contain valuable minerals and vitamins. Alfalfa, burdock root, chamomile, horsetail, oat straw, nettle and red raspberry are all good for general nourishment of the hair, skin and nails.

The following vitamins and minerals that are beneficial for the skin are:

- **25 mg** Zinc
- **10,000 IU** Vitamin A
- **2 gm** Vitamin C
- **100 mg** Vitamin B6

De-Stress

Ringing phones, air pollution, bad news and arguments are just some of the factors that contribute to increased stress levels. Deal with the stress, in any way that will help. These can include meditation, exercise, Tai Chi, or yoga.

Getting out into nature is very important. As Robert Bateman, the famous naturalist says:

> ...if kids play outdoors, not organized sports but unsupervised, climbing trees and building forts, they have less obesity, attention deficit disorder, suicide, alcohol abuse and bullying, and have higher marks. There are movements in progress to redesign areas of cities to have wilderness, not parks, for kids to play on their own. (2009, p. 27)

Get outside and take a walk near the water, or visit your favourite tree. Never underestimate the power of nature to re-charge and renew.

When you need to, call in the stress busters: your friendly Holistic Health Practitioner; try out therapies such as reflexology, massage, aromatherapy, Indian head massage, and Qi stone massage, etc. See what works for you.

Tree Ceremony

Given to me to share with my readers by an Apache medicine woman, the following ceremony is a powerful de-stresser. It seems to help bring down high blood pressure and works on many levels in the body and mind.

Humans and trees have very similar energetic fields and work well together, as what is needed by one is given by the other. For example, humans breathe in oxygen and breathe out carbon dioxide. The trees breathe in carbon dioxide and breathe out oxygen. Trees will take our negative thoughts and transform them. At the end of being with a tree, you will feel replenished and revitalized.

1. Find your favourite tree, take off your shoes and socks (for the brave, do this in all weather conditions) and relax with your back to the tree.

2. Now breathe in deeply, doing the Polarity Breath, become one with the tree and feel yourself developing roots that go into the earth.

3. Now relax into the tree and start to recapitulate your day starting with the most recent events and working backwards.

4. When you feel that you are complete, just simply say thank you to the tree spirits for helping you release the day. This ceremony can be done every night.

Up Your Attitude

Research on optimism concludes that fostering a positive attitude leads to physical and emotional well-being. Take the time to build your optimism and you will find you are more successful in dealing with obstacles that come your way. If you find it difficult, see if you can allow yourself to imagine yourself being more optimistic. More resources can be found in the back of the book.

Get Your Beauty Sleep

Health and beauty, cannot be achieved without quality sleep.

When we do not get sufficient sleep, it results in elevated levels of the hormone cortisol. Even though cortisol is an essential hormone in the body, in excess quantities it has many side effects and. can actually break down tissue. For example, it breaks down muscle tissue, ages our skin, decalcifies our bones, and elevates our blood sugar. When we are sleep-starved, we tend to crave carbohydrates, because cortisol raises blood sugar and insulin levels, unbalancing our system. When we have adequate sleep, we release a "youth" hormone called the human growth hormone. This hormone does exactly the opposite of cortisol – it improves rather than detracts. It results in more youthful body plus increased muscle mass, a healthier skin, and stronger bones.

Essential oils can be of tremendous help here. A nice bath with 6 drops of essential oil (either a single one, or a number of them combined), can help to de-stress the body and mind, and bring peace to the soul. Some relaxing essential oils include Marjoram, Lavender, Chamomile and Ylang ylang. Chamomile also has an anti-inflammatory effect and is frequently used in products for children.

Meditation techniques also help to improve your sleep *(see the next section).*

If you have nightmares, Talbot (2009) believes you may be in a 'dream rut'. Some ways to deal with this are to:

- rehearse more benign scenarios to your nightmare throughout the day

- practice imagining relaxing images while listening to relaxing music, and/or

- write down your dreams and then change them in any way you wish, and then practice bringing the revised dream to mind throughout the day.

As Talbot discusses, dreams may be a powerful symptom that something is amiss, that aspects of your life are too intense. You may wish to reduce the time you spend watching disturbing images on television or in movies and if you have a more sensitive nature, you may wish to take precautions to set clearer boundaries in your life, and guard yourself from disturbances, especially before going to bed.

Sleepy Time Pillow

Upon this pillow lay your head.
Relax your body make it, feel like lead.
Your mind you must let go blank
Don't go thinking of the bank
Take a deep breath and count to ten
Z'hen very slowly let it out again
Repeat five, six times or more
And very soon you will start to snore.

Jacqui Benham

Create flower pillows to gently lull you to sleep, induce dreams, awaken love, or stimulate the senses.

When making flower pillows, take the time to create beautiful covers using velvet, silk, or other soft, natural materials. It takes many dried flowers to make a pillow; so sew them small enough to fill easily. For example: a small two-by-four to a larger size that measures eight inches by twelve inches. I would suggest making an inner lining of muslin to hold the flowers and to stop them from leaking out.

Experiment with the proportions of dried flowers for the scent you want and add a few drops of essential oils for extra aroma.

INGREDIENTS

Foundational Ingredients
>   Dried herbs of: Lavender, Chamomile, Spearmint
>   or peppermint

Essential Oils
>   **5 drops** Lavender
>   **2 drops** Rose

Additional ingredients
>   **1/2 tsp.** powdered orris root
>   **1 small** Herkimer diamond

METHOD:

1. Mix equal measures of the dried herbs.
2. Mix the essential oils and the orris root together; cover with cling film and leave for at least one hour.
3. Mix the dried herbs together; add the above mixture and the Herkimer diamond (wrapped in a soft cloth or cotton batting).
4. Fill the muslin bag and place in the pillow cover.

Have a fragrant sleep, and pleasant flower dreams.

Note: The Herkimer diamond is known as a dreaming crystal.

Cultivate Inner Harmony

Webs of light spin across the Earth
Reaching out the golden threads touch
As the golden glow thickens and encircles
The healing begins.

For those of you on the quest for beauty, it frankly cannot be achieved without inner beauty. Inner beauty requires an inner feeling of serenity which only comes if the "itty bitty shitty committee" is shut up in the mind. I stress again, that you cannot have inner harmony if there is internal dialogue going on. The mind needs training and this is where meditation comes in. Now meditation does not necessarily mean sitting in a lotus position looking holier than thou and feeling terribly spiritual. Of course, if this is what you have to do to close that ego mind, then you have my blessings to go for it.

Meditation can take on many forms as it can be achieved when the ego mind is completely occupied and focused. The mind can be trained. There are many courses that if followed, can help with this process. It does take discipline though and should be performed preferably every day, or at the very least, three times a week for it to be effective.

At the Institute we have a meditation course, where students learn how to meditate in a step by step process.

Robert Bateman comments on his healing approach to dealing with cancer:

> I managed my fear well during the cancer
> procedures...by meditating, and I think about "the
> Now," focusing only on what's happening at exactly
> this moment. I don't worry about the state of the
> world, but take action on those things that I can
> change, knowing what I can't. (2009, p. 27)

I would like to share with you some fundamental basics: focusing and breathing techniques. Plus I recommend the *Tree Ceremony* (see above).

Focusing

Let's start with focusing: In relaxation exercises, focusing eliminates outside disturbances or distractions, allowing the mind and body to direct all of its energy to where it is needed the most.

You may use this energy for solution finding, to stimulate creativity, for healing, or simply to find peace of mind.

The process is much like the focusing of a camera lens, which you adjust until what you desire to capture in the picture becomes clear.

Since we are sensuous creatures; we respond to sensory stimulation from the outside world. Involuntary responses to outside stimuli causes stress to build up in the body. When you are able to "turn down" the volume on your stress response mechanism, either by physical or mental means, you have taken the first step to controlling and reducing the stress factors in your life.

On a physical level, what you are doing is slowing down brain wave activity and changing your response pattern. On a physiological level you are putting the ego to sleep.

The ego is a product of our experiences. It is our self-defence mechanism. If your experiences have for the greater part been negative, then it is likely that your ego will block you from trying something new for fear of being hurt. This could manifest as resistance to relaxation exercises in the form of wandering thoughts, yawning, itching, being physically uncomfortable, and refusing to get comfortable or fidgeting.

In effect what we want to do is reassure the ego that it is safe for it to relinquish control and allow us to effect changes that we consciously deem necessary. One very effective method is to lull the ego to sleep by repeating a word, a tone or a vibration over and over. When the ego has been assured that there will be no excitement or danger, the ego will go quiet. This is part of what occurs in the process of hypnosis.

Another purpose for learning to focus is to achieve discipline. Discipline, repetition and habit are three elements of the process of attaining self-mastery. Loving discipline (determination and support) gives you the strength to use repetition (practice) of techniques that will eventually produce new healthy habits. By modifying or eliminating conditioning, we can eventually create beneficial conscious/ unconscious reactions to stimulus. We are in effect creating a new reality for ourselves.

It is important to find the time and create the space with which to follow any technique that you choose, and then to stick with it. The timetable may be based on natural rhythms (sunrise/sunset) or on imposed ones. Seek your own natural rhythms, taking into account that you may have to deal with years of established conditioning.

Repeat your meditation practice at least three times a week for a minimum of three months and it will become a habit you don't want to break.

Last, but not least, I would like to speak to you about listening to your heart and becoming your true authentic self. In contrast with the inner critic, this is what is known in some circles as your higher self or intuition. Each of us possesses this voice. It guides as, it supports us and it helps us make decisions. By focusing, you can learn to hear this inner voice more clearly. Whether accessed by relaxation, meditation or prayer, this voice is in each individual waiting to be heard.

The action of focusing may be likened to the sun's light. Scattered, it falls all around you providing light, warmth, healing and growth. Focused, it becomes a laser which is able to start a fire, cut through metal or incise a tumour. The power of your mind is like the sun's light. Focused, this energy enables you to become the master, not the victim of your own life.

Focusing agents are words or images, tones or vibrations that serve as a fixed point in our consciousness, unmoving and grounding. By repeating these focusing agents, we slow down brain activity, thus calming the mind and body. The heart is a portable focusing agent that is always with us. Each heart beats in a unique rhythm. By using your own heartbeat as a focusing agent, you will become aware of yourself and your wonderful body.

Focusing on the Universal Heart Rhythm

Now let's practise some focusing techniques: During the following exercise, you will learn to get in touch with your body, by focusing on your very own heart rhythm.

1. Find yourself a comfortable position. Loosen any tight garments and remove anything that might distract you, such as jewellery or glasses. Close your eyes.

2. Start by taking deep, relaxing, abdominal breaths. On each exhalation see the tension that might be in your body released, to help your body you may repeat "relax" to yourself. As you become more relaxed, start to slow your thoughts and clear your mind. Focus inward and listen to any and all noises within your body, for example, your digestive tract, the sound of blood rushing through your veins, arteries and capillaries of your heart.

3. Slowly eliminate all sounds except your heartbeat. Become familiar with the beats and start to count them. After a while, start to breathe in time with your heartbeat.

Inhale.... hold.... exhale. You may use any of the following counts, depending upon the ease and comfort that you feel. Breathe in that rhythm for a while. You may change to a longer or shorter count until you find the one that is yours.

Do not force your breathing.

Breathing patterns

Inhale	2 beats
Hold	1 beat
Exhale	2 beats

Or

Inhale	3 beats
Hold	1 beat
Exhale	3 beats

Or

Inhale	4 beats
Hold	2 heats
Exhale	4 beats

You may use any of the following sequences:

5-2-5	6-3-6	7-3-7
7-4-7	9-4-9	12-5-12

Breathe

Good health, vitality and mental clarity are some of the many beneficial effects of proper breathing. Oxygen serves as a natural painkiller, muscle relaxant, energizer, sensory augmenter and brain food in general. A lack of oxygen results in the death of brain cells.

The action of breathing brings oxygen into the lungs where it is transferred to the bloodstream. This life-giving element along with nutrients is then carried to all organs and the brain via the arteries and returned to the lungs via the veins. Waste products, carbon dioxide (and some germs) are expelled with each exhalation.

Poor posture, bad living habits and poor circulation can rob us of precious oxygen. The body tends to tire and slump after hours of sitting at a desk in an uncomfortable chair or position. The lungs sag down into the diaphragm (our breathing muscle), impeding full expansion of the lungs and thus reducing our oxygen intake. By doing regular breathing exercises you can increase your lung capacity and get more nourishment from the air you breathe.

Lack of sleep, poor diet, smoking, pollution, anxiety, and lack of exercise or restricted movement can contribute to sluggish circulation. Of what use is fuel, if it does not get to the furnace? Practice good living habits to improve circulation. For example, get plenty of rest, good nourishment, do relaxation exercises, practice positive thinking and enjoy regular exercise.

The following exercise can be used to reach a state where you will be open to your inner voice or simply to relax. Once a rhythm is established, let your body breathe for itself and listen. To go deeper, simply say to yourself, "relax and go deeper".

Standing Deep Breathing

Try the following simple movements to counteract the effects of sitting for long periods of time:

1. Regularly stand up and stretch.

2. Now raise your arms upwards, taking a long slow deep breath.

3. Hold the breath for a moment.

4. As you lower your arms, exhale slowly.

5. Repeat this action three times or more if necessary.

6. Nod your head up and down while turning it from side to side.

7. Roll your head from side to side loosely without straining your neck or forcing the movement.

8. Gently, taking your time, raise both your shoulders towards your ears and then slowly lower them to the starting position.

9. Shake your hands loosely from the wrist.

Afterwards, take note of how you feel. Breathe slowly, relaxing your waist. Allow your waistline to expand with each inhalation to contract with each exhalation. Never force your breathing. This kind of breathing is known as abdominal breathing. If your clothes are too tight for this kind of breathing, loosen your belt or waistband. Breathe slowly and gently to avoid hyperventilation.

From here you can create a new reality or simply remember that you are a perfect being... .after a while, start to come back to the here and now. Become aware of your physical body by letting it move whatever part wants to be moved and stretched. Open your eyes when you feel ready to.

....Hi there perfect being....

Polarity Breathing

The following breathing technique is known as polarity breathing. These breaths will balance and calm specific areas of the body.

1. Start by taking several, deep abdominal breaths. Allow your waist to expand as you inhale and contract as you exhale.

2. Start to breathe in through your nose and out through your nose....... Repeat three times. Feel the relaxation spreading at the base of your spine, as your tailbone connects with the ground (or chair).

3. Next breathe in through nose and out through your mouth. Repeat three times. Feel your pelvis relaxing.

4. Now breathe in through your mouth and out through your nose..... Repeat three times. Feel your solar plexus relaxing and expanding.

5. The next breath is in through your mouth and out through your mouth ....
   Repeat three times. Feel your chest relaxing and opening. Feel the warmth spreading around your heart.

6. The next breath is a subtle, gentle breath: loosen your jaw and breathe in through your nose and mouth at the same time... then exhale through your nose and mouth at the same time.... Repeat three times. Feel your throat and neck relaxing and expanding as your breathing passage opens completely.

7. Breathe naturally now into your core.... Let your body breathe for itself and listen to your breath....

8. Open your eyes when you feel ready.

These breathing sequences, fifteen in all can be done anywhere without attracting attention. They can be done with the eyes open or closed, on a bus, at your desk, or even in a public washroom.

> *Remember when you are feeling tense,*
> *take the time to breathe.*

Now for the outer you....

PART
FIVE

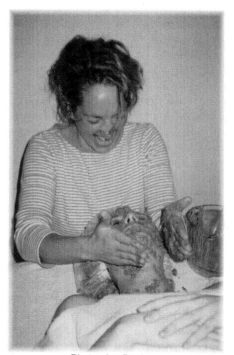

Photo: Jan Benham

Facial Care

Follow the basic skin care routine, making sure that you use the appropriate cleanser, toner and moisturiser.

Basic Skin Care Routine

- In the morning, cleanse the face and neck with the cleansing lotion/cream of your choice. Wipe off excess with damp cotton wool.

- Tone the face by applying the toner with cotton wool.

- Moisturise with the moisturiser of your choice.

- In the evening, do the same as above with the exception of the moisturiser; use a night cream or treatment cream/gel instead.

Note: The ultimate skin boost is to add 1 dollop of natural organic yoghurt to 50 ml of your favourite moisturiser.

Cleansing

It is important to cleanse your face for a smooth, clear and youthful skin. If you wear makeup, then it must first be cleansed or your skin will be prevented from breathing and will clog up, leaving a rather rough texture.

It is important that the cleansing should be done as gently as possible. I do not advocate the use of scrubs on the face as people tend to be too rough and stretch the skin into all sorts of exaggerated states. Remember what your mother said that if the wind changes direction when you are making a face then it will stay in that position. Well, if you keep pulling the skin around, especially the skin around the eyes, then you will have a loose baggy skin!!!

You have to treat the skin of the face differently from the skin on the body. For example, I do not advocate the use of soap on the face as it is too drying and changes the pH balance of the skin. Even on the body, if you want to use soap, try to find a natural soap that has no chemicals, artificial fragrance or colouring in it or check out making your own soap. I recommend pure olive oil soap as it is the gentlest soap in the world. We sell the *Olive Oil Cleansing Cake* at the Aroma shoppe and many people find it beneficial.

To learn how to make your own soaps, see the author's newest book *Successful Soap* (*now in press!*).

As well as daily cleansing, it is essential, and a real treat, once a week, to have a deep cleansing treatment such as a face mask, or a facial steam.

After cleansing, it is important to tone, to rebalance the skin's pH factor, remove any cleanser residue that might be left on the face, and to prepare it for moisturising.

Use an eye-serum or moisturiser that is specially-formulated for the delicate area around your eyes.

Seasonal Refreshing

I recommend having a professional facial done at least four times a year, in line with the four seasons. This is especially important during winter when the skin can become dehydrated from the double whammy of the drying effect of cold winter weather and the central heating we use inside our homes.

Professionals use their knowledge and years of experience to analyze your skin type: sensitive, dry, excessively dry, normal or oily. They can provide valuable insight into how to best care for your skin at home.

Also, regular facials provide a safety check on the level of treatment you give your skin. For example, some people can overdo the tanning bed, or overuse *exfoliants*, or other highly stimulating treatments.

Facials are also the best way to deal with blemishes. For instance, extracting black heads or treating skin eruptions on your own can lead to bruising or broken capillaries, and possibly result in irreversible keloids, scarring and discoloration.

After a facial, your face may be slightly red, and you should refrain from wearing make-up to allow your skin to breathe. Therefore, if you have a big event, it is best to book a facial at least a few days beforehand to allow your skin some recovery time.

Cleansers

Jojoba Cleanser

The following cleansing lotion deeply cleanses the skin, removing all traces of grime and makeup. Use daily, wiping off excess with damp cotton wool and follow with a skin toner and moisturiser. This is suitable for all skin types.

INGREDIENTS:

Waxes and oils:
>   **1 oz (4 dsp)** Lanette emulsifying wax
>   **20 ml (2 dsp)** Fractionated Coconut oil
>   **40 ml (4 dsp)** Jojoba oil

Waters:
>   **600 ml** Distilled water
>   **100 ml** Rose water

Essential Oils:
>   **16 drops** Lavender
>   **8 drops** Rose geranium
>   **3 drops** Palmarosa

Preservatives
>   **1 dollop** Grapefruit seed extract

METHOD:
Follow the *Basic Instructions*.

Note: 1 dollop is a large drop.

Apricot Cleanser

For those of you with dryer skin, the *Apricot Cleanser* might be just what the doctor ordered. The only difference from the *Jojoba Cleanser* is to substitute the Jojoba oil for Apricot kernel oil and to change the essential oil blend.

INGREDIENTS:

Waxes and oils:
    1 oz (4 dsp) Lanette emulsifying wax
    20 ml (2 dsp) Fractionated Coconut oil
    40 ml (4 dsp) Apricot kernel oil
Waters:
    600 ml Distilled water
    100 ml Rose water
Essential Oils:
    14 drops Petitgrain
    10 drops Lavender
    3 drops Neroli
Preservatives
    1 dollop Grapefruit seed extract

METHOD:
Follow the *Basic Instructions*.

Rose Cleansing Cream

For a thicker cleansing cream, this rose cleanser is especially good for the removal of makeup.
Suitable for dry skin.

INGREDIENTS:

Waxes and oils:
   1 tsp. Beeswax
   2 dsp. Shea butter
   1 oz. Lanette wax
   40 ml Apricot kernel oil
   20 ml Fractionated Coconut oil
Waters:
   250 ml Distilled water
   100 ml Rose water
Essential Oils:
   8 drops Rose geranium
   1 drop Rose absolute
Preservative:
   1 dollop Grapefruit seed extract

METHOD:
Follow the *Basic Instructions*.

Honey Cleanser

For those of you that like the feeling of soap on the face. Here is a gentle alternative facial cleanser. This is a mild non-soap cleanser that works well for all skin types.

INGREDIENTS:

¼ **cup** Honey
1 tbsp. *Experimental Basic Shampoo.*
½ **cup** Vegetable glycerin

METHOD:
Heat the honey and gently stir in the glycerin and liquid shampoo, and pour into sterilized bottle.

Toners

Toners rinse away traces of oils and fats (residue from the cleansers); they help to close pores, restore the skin's acid mantle (pH factor), stimulate circulation and refine texture. Use after cleansing and before moisturising.

Rose Geranium Freshener

Suitable for all skin types.

INGREDIENTS:

Foundational Ingredients
    150 ml Distilled water
    90 ml Rose water
    10 ml Witch Hazel
Essential Oils
    5 drops Rose geranium
    4 drops Lavender

METHOD:
Mix the essential oils into the Witch Hazel, "gently shaken, and not stirred". Now simply add the distilled water and rose water and shake again.

This makes for an individual 250 ml size bottle of toner. To make a 1 litre size, simply quadruple the quantities.

Purifying Freshener

Suitable for normal to oily skin.

INGREDIENTS:

Foundational Ingredients
>**150 ml** Distilled water
>**90 ml** Lemon balm water
>**10 ml** Witch Hazel

Essential Oils
>**5 drops** Mandarin
>**3 drops** Juniper berry
>**1 drop** Patchouli

METHOD:

Mix the essential oils into the Witch Hazel, "gently shaken and not stirred". Now simply add the distilled water and Lemon balm water and shake again.

Note: For an instant cooling sensation, add chunks of cucumber to either of the fresheners. Cucumber is great for preventing blemishes while firming and cooling the skin.

Other ingredients that work well in fresheners are Aloe vera and Seaweed extract.

Just add a dollop of either to your favourite freshener.

Moisturisers

Moisturisers are needed to protect and nourish our skin. The wind, sun and central heating, dry out our skin, leaving the skin dryer than it should be. Moisturisers replace the loss of moisture in the skin, even skins that are oily and acneic need moisturising. Moisturise when the skin is moist, after cleansing and toning.

Eye Serum

INGREDIENTS:

7.5 ml Seaweed extract
Essential Oils:
    1 drop Lemon
    1 drop Cypress
    1 drop Lavender

METHOD:
Put a tiny drop of Seaweed extract in the bottom of a 7.5 ml glass eye dropper bottle, add the essential oils, shake and fill up with the Seaweed extract and cap.

Combo Plate Moisturiser

Suitable for all skin types.

INGREDIENTS:

Waxes and oils:
>**1 oz.** Coco palm emulsifying wax
>**40 ml** Jojoba oil
>**20 ml** Fractionated Coconut oil

Waters:
>**250 ml** Distilled water
>**100 ml** Rose water

Preservative:
>**1 dollop** Grapefruit seed extract

Essential Oils:
>**12 drops** Lavender
>**8 drops** Geranium
>**7 drops** Palmarosa

METHOD:
Follow the *Basic Instructions*.

Note: To make a basic white cream, just use the recipe from the combo plate moisturiser without the essential oils.

Soothing Moisturiser

Suitable for sensitive/dry skin.

INGREDIENTS:

Waxes and oils:
>**1 oz.** Coco palm emulsifying wax
>**60 ml** Apricot kernel oil
>**1 dollop** Carrot root oil
>**1 dollop** Vitamin E

Waters:
>**250 ml** Distilled water
>**100 ml** Rose water

Preservative:
>**1 dollop** Grapefruit seed extract

Essential Oils:
>**12 drops** Lavender
>**8 drops** Mandarin
>**4 drops** Palmarosa
>**3 drops** Roman chamomile
>**3 drops** Sandalwood

METHOD:
Follow the *Basic Instructions.*

La Jeunesse Night Cream

Suitable for dry skin.

INGREDIENTS:

Waxes and oils:
      1 oz. Coco palm emulsifying wax
      1 tsp. Beeswax
      1 tsp. Shea butter
      60 ml Jojoba oil
      20 ml Apricot kernel oil
      1 dollop Vitamin E
Waters:
      250 ml Distilled water
      100 ml Orange blossom water
Preservative:
      1 dollop Grapefruit seed extract
Essential Oils:
      9 drops Bergamot
      4 drops Sandalwood
      3 drops Frankincense
      2 drops Jasmine absolute

METHOD:
Follow the *Basic Instructions*.

Ultra-Firming Gel

This gel refines, moisturises and tightens the skin as it repairs. It also helps to control excess oil and the build-up of sebum on the skin. Good for all skin types, especially for ageing skin. Use as a night treatment.

INGREDIENTS:

Gel:
> **50 ml** Seaweed gel

Essential Oils:
> **15 drops** Cypress
> **10 drops** Clary sage
> **2 drops** Frankincense

METHOD:
Add the essential oils into the seaweed gel, stir and pour into a sterilized jar.

Masks, Facials and Fruit Facials

There are a lot of great masks on the market. One of my favourites is Dead sea mud and French Green Clay mixed with rose water. I find that it is good for skin problems ranging from eczema, psoriasis, acne, dry and oily skin, to name just a few. Most manufacturers suggest letting the mask completely dry, but I personally prefer to cover the mask with cling film, leaving it on for 15 minutes then removing it with a hot damp towel (try not to ruin your white towels here but choose a dark colour specifically for your masks). Follow with toner and moisturiser.

Whilst this book was in the final stages of being written, I was teaching an advanced skin care class. In this class, we had tremendous fun playing with fruits and vegetables on the skin. We massaged our skin with honey and treated our skin to a cornucopia of strawberries, cucumber, eggs, bananas and avocados. The benefits were incredible and I ended up incorporating them into all the treatments at my clinic.

The clients and students loved it so much that I decided to complete the facial care section with a special discussion of the merits of fruits and foods on the skin.

Fruit facials go well with the previous treatments mentioned in this book, and blend well with essential oils adding a special signature touch to your facial routine.

A mortar and pestle is very useful for mashing the fruit for fruit facials.

Aromatherapy Steam Facial

Aromatherapy steam facials open the pores and help to push out dirt and impurities, at the same time they help to heal blemishes.

INGREDIENTS:

Foundational ingredient:
Boiling water *(enough to fill a large bowl).*
Essential Oils:
4 – 6 drops combined
The following essential oils can be either used singularly or combined. They can also be added to the solid masks with the same effect.

For cleansing, use Lavender, Geranium, Tea tree and Rosemary.

For baby boomer tightening: Use cypress, fennel, carrot seed, peppermint and clary sage.

METHOD:
Pour boiling water into a bowl and add your favourite essential oil(s).

TO APPLY:

- Pour the boiling water into the bowl and add the essential oils.

- Make a towel into a head tent and steam the face over the bowl for ten minutes.

- Blot dry, tone and moisturise.

Honey Massage

This is stimulating and cleansing to the skin, good for ageing older skins, especially for heavy smokers and those with heavy wrinkles, or sun damaged thick skin.

INGREDIENTS:

Foundational ingredient:
>   **5 ml** of *Experimental Basic Lotion*

Fruit or food:
>   **5 ml** Honey.

METHOD:
Mix the lotion and honey together.

TO APPLY:

1. This massage is ideally done after steaming the face and is performed for not more than ten minutes.

2. Apply the Honey Massage mixture to the face and neck, massaging in an upward and outward movement starting with the neck first.

3. When the mix starts to feel sticky, and you are unable to massage any more, tap with fingertips quickly on the skin, and remove with damp cotton pads.

Papaya Facial

Using papaya or pineapple removes dead skin cells through the enzymatic action. The skin will look younger and feel smoother when the dead skin layers have been removed. Be careful not to leave the fruit on for too long as they can be extremely drying. Do not leave on for longer than five minutes.

INGREDIENTS

2 tbsp. mashed Papaya or Pineapple
1 tsp. Aloe vera gel

METHOD:

Mix the Papaya and Aloe vera to make a smooth paste. Alternately, simply place gauze pads in the juice and leave to soak for 5 minutes.

TO APPLY:

- After cleansing and toning, apply to face and neck and let sit for a maximum of 5 minutes.

- Rinse with cool water, tone and moisturise.

Note: For an added treat, place slices of cucumber on the eyes while your fruit facial is on.

Strawberries & Cream Facial

This mask is good for dry skin, softens fine wrinkles, and improves tone and texture of the skin.

INGREDIENTS

> **1 large** strawberry mashed (remove the stem)
> **1 tsp.** heavy cream (35% preferred).

METHOD:

Mix the ingredients to make a smooth paste.

TO APPLY:

- After cleansing and toning, apply to the face and leave on for 10-20 minutes.

- Rinse with cool water, tone and moisturise.

Banana Facial

Contains potassium and other nutrients that nourish the skin, leaving it feeling silky and soft. This mask is food for dry skin.

INGREDIENTS

1 banana mashed
2 tsp. apricot kernel oil
1 egg yolk (separate from the white)

METHOD:
Mix the ingredients to make a smooth paste.

TO APPLY:

- After cleansing and toning, apply to the face and leave on for 20 minutes.

- Rinse with cool water, tone and moisturise.

Avocado Facial

This mask is great for tired and mature skin. In Aromatherapy, we use avocado oil in treatments to help with dry skin. Avocado contains both saturated and mono-saturated fatty acids with relatively large amounts of vitamins A, B and D. Its healing properties help to regenerate cells. This facial is useful in the healing of scarred tissue and ageing skin. Avocado also helps to soothe eczema.

INGREDIENTS
>**1** Avocado mashed
>**1 tsp.** clear Honey
>**1 tsp.** plain natural Yogurt
>**2 drops** of Lemon essential oil <u>or</u> **1 tsp.** of lemon juice

METHOD:
Mix the ingredients to make a smooth paste.

TO APPLY:
- After cleansing and toning, apply to the face and leave on for 30 minutes.

- Rinse with cool water, tone and moisturise.

Getting creative:
More Fruit Masks and Treatments

Fruits and vegetables can be used alone, mixed or combined with a thickener.

INGREDIENTS:

Fruit or food:
>Most fruits or other foods can be used in a facial. *The next page has more specific information.*
>Fruit or vegetable is mashed up.

Thickener:
>If the mixture is too runny, it can be thickened by adding a little of one of the following ingredients: honey, raw oatmeal, French green clay, kaolin, mashed banana, whipped egg white or yogurt.

Thinners
>Add milk if the mixture is too thick.

Acidic substances:
>To make a slightly acid mantle, add a few drops of Apple Cider vinegar or Lemon juice.

Moisturising agents
>If the skin is dry, add **one tbsp.** of oil – apricot kernel, avocado, sweet almond or calendula.

Essential Oils:
>For a more powerful treatment add **3 drops** of essential oil(s). (See *Aromatherapy Steam Facial* above).

METHOD:

Mash the fruit, add oils, acidic substances and essential oils. (See the specific instructions for each item below).

Favourite skin foods

Please note; you should not put anything on your skin that you would not eat. In skin care, my favourite "skin friendly" foods do the following:

Apple
A slice of apple lightens dark circles under the eyes.

Avocado
In aromatherapy massage, we use avocado oil to relieve dry skin. Avocado contains both saturated and mono-saturated fatty acids with relatively large amounts of vitamins A, B and D. Their healing properties help to regenerate cells and are useful in the healing of scarred tissue and ageing skin. Avocado also helps to soothe eczema. Mash, and add binder (thickener) if desired.

Banana
Mash and apply.

Carrots
Carrot root oil is an antioxidant, rich in beta-carotene, vitamins B, C, D, and E. It also contains essential fatty acids. This oil is especially good for dry, chapped skin and has rejuvenating properties, delaying the ageing process of the skin. Just add a dollop to any of the fruits.

Carrot seed essential oil
This is another story. This essential oil is known to help with mature, ageing skin, wrinkles, psoriasis and eczema. One drop is all that is needed to be added to a mask or a cream.

Cranberries
If the appearance of freckles on your skin bothers you, crush fresh cranberries and rub into the skin. Leave on for five minutes.

Cucumber Cools and firms the skin making this a great addition to cleansers and toners. Mash, and add binder if desired. Slices of cucumber make great eye pads.

Egg white Firms and tones the skin. Whisk until stiff and brush on: 1/4 tsp. of Cider vinegar may be added to balance the acid mantle of the skin. Alternatively, whisk the egg white with 1 tbsp. of milk.

Egg yolk Adds proteins and vitamins to the skin. Beat and combine with 1 tbsp. of honey and 1 tsp. of any carrier oil.

Honey Put a dot of honey on an inflamed pimple to draw it out.

Papaya Enzymatic action helps clear away dead-cell debris. These enzymes are known as *papain* and seem to digest dead cell debris on the skin. Soak gauze pads in the juice and leave on the skin for 5 minutes.

Pineapple Enzymatic action helps clear away dead-cell debris. These enzymes are known as *bomelain* and seem to digest undesirable stuff on the skin. Soak gauze pads in the juice and leave on the skin for 20 minutes?.

Strawberry When freshly mashed and applied, this softens and lightens the skin and helps balance the pH factor. Mix with oatmeal if too sloppy to work with.

Yogurt Cleanses, tones and extracts. Can be used alone or with other ingredients. Also useful in reducing the appearance of freckles.

Special Treatments

There are three common themes among baby boomers that I have come across in my practice as a Holistic Health Practitioner:

- Ageing skin *(this may include slackening, sagging or thickening of the skin)*

- Congested skin, large pores, spots or acne

- Sensitive, Reddened Skin

With each problem, I have formulated appropriate day-to-day care, plus treatments that can be done at home or in a clinic, with a trained holistic skin care specialist. Let's begin with ageing!

The Ageing Process

For all you baby boomers out there....

The inner dermal layer is composed of connective tissue, primarily protein fibres – **elastin** and **collagen**. Elastin provides elasticity to the skin; that gives the qualities of stretch and the ability to return to its original shape and form. Collagen gives the skin its tone and strength.

Why do elastin and collagen have a special mention?

Well, these protein fibres play an important role in how fast we age. If we let those free radicals get out of control by not eating the right foods, drinking enough water, and exercising, then damage occurs throughout the body affecting the skin (especially for some reason on the face and neck), causing it to sag as it begins to lose its natural elasticity and wrinkle as the collagen fibres start to become twisted and matted.

The good news is that we can slow down the effects of ageing and can even repair some of the damage that has already occurred.

In my clinic, we have had great success with our neck firming treatments and our anti-ageing facials. So included in our special treatment section is a step-by-step guide on how to perform your own treatments.

How the skin ages:

Age 20   The facial skin is free of wrinkles.

Age 25   First wrinkles appear on the forehead and under eyes – laugh lines show up.

Age 30   Crow's feet appear at the corner of the eyes.

Age 40   Permanent wrinkles appear from ears to neck.

Age 45   Eyes become more sunken, double chin may appear, lips become thinner and eyebrows more bushy.

Age 50   Wrinkles appear around the nose, earlobes and chin. Skin becomes more noticeably dry.

Age 55	Folds form at nape of neck and hyper pigmentation or skin discolouration appears on areas exposed to sunlight.
Age 60	Wrinkles around mouth deepen and cheeks begin to sag.
Age 70	Wrinkles begin to overlap, scalp hair becomes thinner and pigmentation now becomes quite evident.

All is not lost though; ageing of the skin can be slowed down and even reversed to a certain extent. Yes, miracles do happen! We have had tremendous results at the clinic.

Just follow the instructions in this book,
to give you a brand new look.

The number one enemy of the skin and primary cause of ageing is damage caused by free radicals as discussed earlier. Ageing is also affected by the food we eat, poor circulation, dehydration of cells and cellular intoxication.

For more information about dealing with these, see the 'Inner Care' section.

How do we deal with this?

Every night cleanse with the *Rose Cleansing Cream*, tone with the *Rose Geranium Freshener*, and apply the *La Jeunesse Night Cream*. In the morning, use the *Jojoba Cleansing Lotion*, tone with the *Rose Geranium Freshener* and moisturise with the *Ultra-Firming Gel* on the face and neck, and the *Eye Serum* around the eyes.

Poor circulation, poor nutrition, and over-exposure of the skin to the sun can, over time, contribute to needless wrinkles, or even the thickening of the skin (or leather-like skin). For people who have premature ageing, use the *Fruit Acid Lotion* every evening as a night treatment and moisturise in the morning with the *Ultra-Firming Gel*.

For sagging skin, do the *Neck Firming Exercise* daily and complete the *Rejuvenating and Firming Treatment* at least once per month to maintain youthful skin.

For more intensive healing, follow the complete course of the *Rejuvenating and Firming Treatment*.

Neck Firming Exercise

This exercise firms the skin around the jaw line and the neck. First, gently create a circle with your shoulders (up to your ears, back, down,-forward and back) to relax them. Do this three times. Then bring your shoulders up, back and down again, leaving them in this position while you gently arch the head back. Then try to touch the tip of your nose with the tip of your tongue and hold for three seconds (do the tongue stretch ten times).

Eye Treatment

For firming the eye area – soak eye pads with Witch Hazel mixed with 1 drop each of Cypress, Lavender and Frankincense and leave for 15 minutes.

Rejuvenating & Firming Treatment

At least twice a year, do the following rejuvenating and firming treatment.

Complete this treatment 3 times per week for 3 weeks then reduce to once a week for 3 weeks more, for a total of 12 treatments twice a year. The following two recipes are used in this treatment.

Compress
INGREDIENTS:

Foundational Ingredient:
>   **50 ml** *Rose Geranium Freshener*

Essential Oils:
>   **3 drops** Clary sage
>   **3 drops** Cypress
>   **1 drop** Frankincense

>   Gauze or "man-strength" tissues

METHOD:
Mix the essential oils into the *Rose Geranium Freshener*

Rejuvenating and Firming Cream

INGREDIENTS:

Foundational Ingredient:
>   **1 tsp. (5 ml)** *Experimental Basic Cream*

Essential Oils:
>   **3 drops** Fennel
>   **3 drops** Cypress
>   **1 drop** Carrot seed *(not oil)*

METHOD:
Place the cream in a bowl. Add the essential oils and mix.

Treatment Process
TO APPLY:

1. Cleanse and tone the skin

2. Soak the gauze or tissue into the compress blend.

3. Apply *Compress* on the area of the skin that needs attention, particularly the neck and lower face. Avoid the eye area.

4. Leaving the compress on, steam the area with a facial steamer or use hot wet towels for 15 minutes.

5. Remove the compress and massage the *Rejuvenating and Firming Cream* into the skin in an upward and outwards movement until it is fully absorbed.

6. Tone the face.

7. Apply *Ultra-Firming Gel* to the whole face and neck.

8. On a day-to-day basis, every morning cleanse, tone and moisturise as per your skin type. Every evening after cleansing and toning, apply the *Ultra-Firming Gel* on the face and neck, and the eye serum around the eyes.

Tip: If your skin is "leathered" or damaged due to overexposure to the sun, then use the *Fruit Acid Lotion* as a night treatment for a few weeks to naturally exfoliate the skin before applying the treatment.

Tip: Add the Eye treatment as an added benefit.

Spotty, Congested Skin

This is characterized by the presence of congestion, zits and blackheads (whoever thought that we would still be suffering teenage acne at 40 years old?). Zits and blackhead are mainly seen on the forehead, nose and chin, the *T-zone*. Even when pores are only slightly blocked, this congestion needs to be removed regularly to ensure the flow of oxygen to the skin.

The worst thing that you can do is to use products that contain alcohol. This dries out the skin and, as a result, the sebaceous glands in the skin respond by producing more oil, causing a vicious cycle of oily flaky skin.

How do we deal with this?

Follow the *Basic Skin Care Routine* making sure that you use the appropriate cleanser, toner and moisturiser. For a few weeks it would be good to replace the moisturiser with the *Fruit Acid Lotion* - especially if there is previous acne scarring on the face.

Some suggestions:

Watch the junk food intake and your diet in general. For additional information on an alkaline acid balance diet, see the author's book *The Creamy Craft of Cosmetic Making*.

It is important that any blackheads be removed by a professional therapist on a regular basis so that a build up does not occur. A facial from a holistic skin care specialist given once a week for six weeks would be of incredible value in the healing of the skin, with follow-up treatments once every month. Alternatively, do the *Zit Zapper Treatment* once a week for six weeks.

Tip: Zapping those outbreaks
On zits and inflamed spots, apply 1 drop of Lavender essential oil directly to the spot and leave overnight. Results guaranteed.

Zit Zapper Treatment

1. Cleanse and tone.
2. Steam with a facial steamer for 15 minutes. If you do not have a facial steamer, do an *Aromatherapy Steam Facial* with 2 drops each of Lavender and Tea tree essential oil.
3. If you really must remove your own blackheads (perhaps you're living on an island in the middle of the Pacific Ocean?), be very careful. [Use tissues over fingertips and do not force the extraction as scarring, bruising or even broken (red) capillaries can occur easily that over time will build up and become more noticeable. Some people even develop keloids or skin discoloration. If bleeding does occur, apply a drop of German chamomile essential oil neat to the area. If there is any infection present, watch that is not spread to other areas of the face.] Preferably go to a professional skin care specialist for this part of the facial.
4. Apply a facial clay mask (such as *French Green* or *Fuller's Earth*) mixed with rose water and 3 drops of Lavender essential oil. Leave on for 15 minutes.
5. Remove the mask with a warm wet towel.
6. Tone and moisturise.

Fruit Acid Lotion

Fruit acids gently exfoliate and smooth the skin. There is also some evidence that they stimulate skin repair.

INGREDIENTS

Foundational ingredient:
    15 ml of the *Experimental Basic Lotion*
Essential Oils
    6 drops Grapefruit
    6 drops Lemon
    6 drops Bergamot

METHOD:
Add the essential oils to the lotion. Shake to combine.

TO APPLY:
Use after cleansing and toning, twice daily; some tingling may be felt due to the working action on the skin.

Sensitive, Reddened Skin

Often described as rosacea, this can become a chronic inflammatory condition which mainly affects the nose and cheeks.

Contrary to popular beliefs, I find that the skin is usually very congested, causing the inflammatory effect. Imagine have a splinter in your finger; well, that is exactly what is happening to the skin.

So before the skin can heal, the 'splinter' has to be removed. Afterwards, massage the skin with the appropriate essential oil treatment blend. This can aid in healing of the skin.

Rosacea seems to run in families and shows up usually on people who have sensitive, fair skin.

How do we deal with this?

Follow the *Basic Skin Care Routine*, making sure that you use the appropriate cleanser, toner and moisturiser.

In extreme cases, do the *Rosacea Treatment* once a week for a month.

Diet does help and, it is suggested that one avoid spicy foods and red wine.

Note: Rosacea and sensitive skin often have broken capillaries showing on the nose and cheeks. These can be removed by a professional electrologist who has specialized training in red vein removal.

Rosacea Treatment

To soothe and relax the skin, complete this treatment at least once a week for a month.

Soothing Massage Oil
INGREDIENTS

Foundational ingredient:
    1 dollop Jojoba oil
Essential Oils
    2 drops Lavender
    1 drop German chamomile
    1 drop Neroli
    1 drop Cypress

METHOD:

Add the essential oils to the jojoba oil.

TO APPLY:

- Cleanse and tone.

- Steam with a facial steamer for a maximum of 5 minutes (or as soon as the skin starts to go red). If you do not have a facial steamer, do an *Aromatherapy Steam Facial* with 4 drops of Lavender essential oil.

- Remove the congestion. Note: this should *only* be done by a professional.

- Tone.

- Massage the infected area with the *Soothing Massage Oil* for two minutes.

Note: always massage the skin in an outward direction (as depicted).

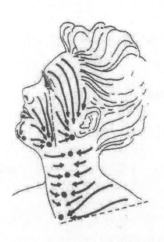

PART SIX

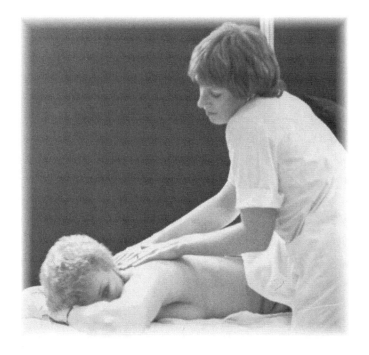

Body Care

You do not have to have 3 sizes of jeans in your closet. No, you are not eighteen years old, but yes, we can change our bodies. All it takes is a little discipline, love and acceptance. To change what we can and to love and accept what we can't change. Our bodies respond to how we think and feel. It is important though to love ourselves for who we are right now and to take one step at a time.

To starve ourselves or over-exercise is just going to make us look tired or exhausted.

We can do things gently through a healthy diet, caring for our skin and exercise is of course important – especially sweating. Just walking (daily), swimming, running, joining a yoga class 3 times a week, will do wonders for your body and health.

Our skin is the largest organ in our bodies. It flushes toxins outward and absorbs nutrients and vitamins from the air and sunlight. A healthy skin expels at least one pound of waste products daily, and works to cleanse the blood and free the system of toxins (see introductory chapter).

Body Treatments

Skin Brushing

One way of helping the body's natural process is through skin brushing with a natural bristle brush. Skin brushing stimulates the circulation, lymphatic system, and has a powerful rejuvenating effect on the nervous system. The major lymph nodes are dumping stations for waste fluids, and, you can stimulate the expulsion of mucoid lymphatic material or impacted lymph (cellulite) by skin brushing. Also, skin brushing removes dead skin layers and other impurities, thus keeping the pores open and unclogged.

To Apply:

Skin brush for a maximum of 5 minutes. This is done dry before bathing. Brush in upward movements towards the heart, with the exception of the abdomen which is brushed down towards the groin (see diagram).

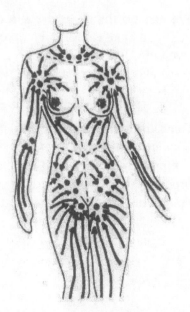

Avoid the face, neck and breasts

After skin brushing, remove the dead skin cells by showering or bathing.

An alternative to skin brushing is to use the orange salt scrub below.

Orange Salt Scrub

This Salt Scrub is effective in stimulating the skin's natural renewal process.

INGREDIENTS

Foundational Ingredients
>**1 cup** Sea salt (fine sea salt) (for an alternative grain, use sugar)
>**1 tsp.** Orange peel powder
>**50 ml** Apricot Kernel oil
>**1 dollop** Vitamin E

Essential Oil
>**10 drops** Orange essential oil

METHOD:
1. Mix the Sea salt and Orange peel powder together.
2. Blend the Apricot kernel oil, vitamin E and orange essential oil together.
3. Mix the oil blend completely into the salt, and put into a sterilized glass jar.

TO APPLY:

- Dampen skin.
- Take a small amount of the scrub, massage on the body. Avoid the face and neck.
- Rinse.

See-You-Later-Alligator Oil Treatment

For the softest, smoothest skin.

INGREDIENTS

Foundational ingredients
    100 ml Apricot Kernel Oil
    1 dollop Vitamin E
Essential Oils
    7 drops Grapefruit
    4 drops Lavender
    1 drop Sandalwood

METHOD:
1. Pour the Apricot kernel oil and Vitamin E into a glass bottle.
2. Add the essential oils and shake gently.

TO APPLY:

- Massage at least 20 ml of the oil into the skin before stepping into a hot bath or shower.

- Allow the heat of the water to push the oil into the skin.

- Do not use soap.

- Afterwards just pat dry.

- For a double whammy, give yourself a course of skin brushing first, and then apply the oil before bathing.

In-a-While-Crocodile Bath

Algae is a powerful detoxifier and seems to act as a magnet to all toxins and debris lurking in the skin. Algae is also valuable in treating muscular and joint conditions. For an individual bath, blend the following ingredients:

INGREDIENTS

Foundational ingredient
　　1 oz. (2 tbsp.) of algae powder
Essential Oils
　　4 drops Juniper berry
　　3 drops Grapefruit
　　2 drops Rosemary

METHOD:
Mix the algae powder with the essential oils.

TO APPLY:
- Pour the entire mixture into a warm running bath.

- Place a vase of flowers where you can see them, surround your bath with small scented votive candles, dim the lights and add meditative music.

- Soak in the bath for a minimum of 15 minutes.

Body Washes

Luxurious Body Wash

This is a great body wash that is made with organic products, and is free of parabens, petroleum or artificial dyes, and yet it provides a luxurious and sensuous feeling.

INGREDIENTS

250 ml Rose water
1 pinch Citric Acid
1/2 tsp. Xanthan Gum
1 dollop Vegetable glycerin
125 ml Cornacopa
1 dollop Wheat protein

METHOD:

1. Mix Rose water and Citric acid into a bowl.
2. Sprinkle Xanthan Gum into the bowl, cover and leave overnight.
3. Heat up the mixture and gently mix in the glycerin, Wheat protein and Cornacopa.
4. Pour into a sterilized bottle.

Morning Glow

For a fresh start to your morning, use this invigorating body wash.

INGREDIENTS:

Essential Oils:
>   **6 drops** Rosemary
>   **5 drops** Grapefruit
>   **1 drop** Lavender

METHOD:
To the *Luxurious Body Wash* recipe, add the above ingredients.

Afternoon Delight

This body wash also doubles as a natural bubble bath; just add 2 tsp. to running water.

INGREDIENTS

Essential Oils
>   **8 drops** Bergamot
>   **5 drops** Jasmine
>   **4 drops** Clary sage
>   **2 drops** Sandalwood

METHOD:
To the *Luxurious Body Wash* recipe, add the above ingredients.

Sleep Easy

This body wash helps you to relax and have a good night's sleep.

INGREDIENTS

Essential Oils
>**6 drops** Marjoram
>**8 drops** Lavender
>**4 drops** Ylang ylang

METHOD:

To the *Luxurious Body Wash* recipe, add the above ingredients.

ADDED PLEASURE:

- Place a bowl of Lavender in your room to allow the scent to permeate the space.

- In winter time, add a hot water bottle to warm the bed before you lie down.

Lavender Bath Bomb

The best way to relax after a long stressful day is to have a nice warm bath with a Lavender bath bomb and have a good long soak. The soothing Lavender aroma enchants your senses and gives you a space away from your worries.

INGREDIENTS

Foundational ingredients
> **1/2 tsp.** powdered Orris root
> **1-2 tbsp.** dried flowers such as rosebuds
> **1 cup** Citric acid
> **1 1/8**th cup Baking soda
> **1 tsp.** Fractionated Coconut oil
> **Spray** of Witch Hazel or water

Essential Oil
> **15 drops** Lavender

Colourants
> **1 tsp.** Spirulina or coloured clays

METHOD:

1. Mix the Orris root and dried flowers with the Lavender essential oil. Cover with cling film wrap and leave for at least one hour.
2. Mix the citric acid and baking soda together, add to the above mixture.
3. Slowly add the fractionated Coconut oil, constantly mixing with your hands.
4. Spray with Witch Hazel or water until the mix clumps together.
5. Press into moulds.
6. Release from the mould one hour later

Body Lotions

Exotic Jasmine Body Lotion

Jasmine, known as the "king of flowers", is famous for its aphrodisiac powers. Long used in skin care for dry, sensitive or mature skin, this lotion absorbs quickly into the skin leaving the skin soft and lightly fragranced.

INGREDIENTS

Wax and oils:
  1 oz. Lanette wax
  5 ml (1 tsp.) Shea butter
  60 ml Fractionated Coconut oil
Waters:
  100 ml Jasmine water
  600 ml Distilled water
Essential Oil
  10 drops Jasmine absolute
Preservative
  1 dollop Grapefruit seed extract

METHOD:
Follow the *Basic Instructions*.

Orange Blossom Body Lotion

Neroli essential oil is very soothing: it was reputedly used to calm the nerves of young couples before they engaged in sexual activity. It has the special property of stimulating the growth of healthy new cells, with certain special rejuvenating effects. It can be used for all skin types, but is perhaps most useful for dry or sensitive skins.

INGREDIENTS

Wax and oils:
> **1 oz.** Lanette wax
> **1 tsp. (5 ml)** Shea butter
> **60 ml** Jojoba oil
> **1 dollop** Carrot root oil
> **1 dollop** Vitamin E

Waters:
> **100 ml** Orange blossom water
> **600 ml** Distilled water

Essential Oils:
> **10 drops** Neroli
> **6 drops** Petitgrain

Preservative:
> **1 dollop** Grapefruit seed extract

METHOD:
Follow the *Basic Instructions.*

Nourishing Body Lotion

This nourishing body lotion is designed to offer immediate relief from dry skin, as well as provide long-lasting nourishment. People with very dry skin often experience feelings of discomfort, irritation, lack of suppleness, or they simply notice a coarse, rough appearance to their skin.

INGREDIENTS

Waxes and oils:
>**1 oz.** Lanette wax
>**1 tsp.** Beeswax
>**5 ml** Shea butter
>**50 ml** Apricot kernel oil
>**10 ml** Macadamia nut oil
>**10 ml** Avocado oil
>**1 dollop** Carrot root oil
>**1 dollop** Vitamin E

Waters:
>**100 ml** Rose water
>**650 ml** Distilled water

Essential Oils:
>**7 drops** Mandarin
>**6 drops** Lavender
>**3 drops** Linden blossom absolute

Preservative
>**1 dollop** Grapefruit seed extract

METHOD:
Follow the *Basic Instructions*.

TO APPLY:
Apply liberally twice daily on the body where there is dry skin until relief is achieved.

Body Re-sculpting Oil

This oil provides body re-sculpting action with anti-cellulite results. The essential oils of grapefruit, juniper berry and rosemary help to eliminate toxins and excess fluid. Cypress essential oil stimulates the skin and tones the silhouette. It prevents dehydration, leaving skin supple and satin-smooth.

INGREDIENTS

Foundational Ingredient
        50 ml Apricot kernel oil
Essential Oils:
        12 drops Grapefruit
        6 drops Cypress
        8 drops Rosemary
        4 drops Juniper berry
Preservative
        1 dollop Vitamin E

METHOD:
Place the Apricot kernel oil in a container; add the essential oils and the Vitamin E. Shake.

TO APPLY:
Apply liberally twice daily to areas of the body where cellulite appears.

Hand Care

As we grow older, the skin on the hands becomes dry and loose, exposing the veins. Any fat that once plumped up the skin on the back of the hands lessens. So it is important to use a good moisturising hand cream, and apply often to the hands, paying special attention to the fragile skin on the back.

Like your face, hands are exposed all year round to UV rays, age spots and sunspots (sometimes called liver spots) often appear. Keep your hands protected from the sun's rays. For sun protection apply the *Gardener's Hand Cream* as the sesame and carrot root oils provide good sun screen and protect from the sun's damaging rays (sun protection factor of four).

Our hands are in the water more than we realize: frequent washing, washing dishes, bathing babies, washing our hair, doing laundry, etc., often in irritating detergents. This is unavoidable, yet water quickly dries out the thin skin of our hands by removing the natural oils, prematurely ageing our hands. Wear rubber gloves whenever you can.

Note: If you leave out the wheat protein from the hair shampoo recipe, it can be used as dish washing soap instead of commercially available products. This provides a gentle alternative to using harmful irritating chemicals.

Healthy Nails Oil

This easy-to-use oil goes deep down to support the development of healthy nail beds and helps encourage healthy nail growth with improved nail quality.

INGREDIENTS

Oils:
    7 ml Sweet Almond Oil
    1 dollop Vitamin E
    1 dollop Wheatgerm Oil
Essential Oils:
    4 drops Lavender
    3 drops Lemon
    1 drop Rosemary

METHOD:

1. Mix the oils and Vitamin E together.

2. Add the essential oils to the oil blend.

TO APPLY:

- Massage a drop of the above blend into the cuticles daily.
- This treatment can also be used on the toenails.

Gardener's Hand Cream

This cream is not just for gardening, but for anytime that your hands need tender loving care. It will protect and heal the skin, giving it that smooth and soft feeling.

INGREDIENTS

Waxes and oils:
> **5 ml** Shea butter
> **1 oz.** Lanette wax
> **60 ml** Sesame oil
> **1 dollop** Carrot root oil
> **1 dollop** Vitamin E

Waters:
> **300 ml** Distilled water
> **50 ml** Rose water

Essential Oils:
> **5 drops** Rosemary
> **5 drops** Rose geranium
> **1 dollop** Benzoin
> **2 drops** Myrrh

Preservative:
> **1 dollop** Grapefruit seed extract

METHOD:
Follow the *Basic Instructions.*

TO APPLY:
- Massage into the hands daily as needed.

Lip Care

For luscious kissable lips, try these formulas.

Spearmint Lip Balm

The healing properties of this lip balm help to protect your lips and keep them healthy and smooth.

INGREDIENTS

Waxes and Oils:
>**½ oz.** Beeswax
>**2 tsp.** Shea butter
>**20 ml** Sesame oil
>**60 ml** Apricot kernel oil
>**1 dollop** Carrot root oil
>**1 dollop** Vitamin E

Essential Oils:
>**30 drops** Spearmint
>**5 drops** Myrrh

METHOD:
1. Melt the beeswax, shea butter, sesame and apricot kernel oils in a double boiler.
2. When it is almost melted, add the carrot root oil and Vitamin E stirring all the time.
3. When the waxes and oils are completely melted, remove from the heat.
4. Add the essential oils, immediately pour into sterilized jars.

Chocolate Kisses Lip Balm

This delicious lip balm soothes and protects your lips, whilst also adding a little colour. Have a little fun, and indulge your chocolate addiction.

INGREDIENTS

Waxes and oils:
    ½ oz. Beeswax
    2 tsp. Cocoa butter
    ½ oz. Dark Chocolate (use 78% cacao if possible)
    20 ml Sesame oil
    60 ml Apricot kernel oil
    1 dollop Vitamin E

Essential Oils:
    20 drops Spearmint
    15 drops Sweet Orange

METHOD:

1. Melt the beeswax, cocoa butter, and chocolate, in a double boiler.
2. When it is almost melted, add the sesame, apricot kernel oils and Vitamin E, stirring all the time.
3. When the waxes and oils are completely melted, remove from the heat.
4. Add the essential oils and immediately pour into sterilized jars.

Anti-Viral Lip Balm

The essential oils in this lip balm helps protect and nourish the lips whilst assisting in the healing and prevention of cold sores.

INGREDIENTS

Waxes and Oils:
> **½ oz.** Beeswax
> **2 tsp.** Shea butter
> **20 ml** Sesame oil
> **60 ml** Apricot kernel oil
> **1 dollop** Carrot root oil
> **1 dollop** Vitamin E

Essential Oils:
> **15 drops** Ravensara
> **10 drops** Spearmint
> **5 drops** Tea tree
> **5 drops** Myrrh

METHOD:

1. Melt the beeswax, shea butter, sesame and apricot kernel oils in a double boiler.
2. When it is almost melted, add the carrot root oil and Vitamin E stirring all the time.
3. When the waxes and oils are completely melted, remove from the heat.
4. Add the essential oils, immediately pour into sterilized jars.

Cold Sore Blend

The components of this blend work together to fight off cold sores: bergamot essential oil is known for its powerful anti-viral properties; the vodka dries up the cold sore; and the Lavender essential oil helps in healing of the skin while helping to reduce any possible scarring.

INGREDIENTS

Foundational Ingredient:
    50 drops Vodka
Essential Oils:
    50 drops Bergamot
    50 drops Lavender

METHOD:
Into a 7.5 ml glass eye dropper bottle, mix equal parts (approximately 1/3 each) of the ingredients above.

TO APPLY:
   • Apply neat to the area when tingling is felt

Foot Care

Foot Fixer Cream

This cream will improve the circulation to the feet and calves, and thus help to prevent any aches and pains.

INGREDIENTS

Waxes and oils:
    1 dsp. Beeswax   **20 ml** Calendula oil
    30 ml Shea butter   **40 ml** Avocado oil
    1 oz. Lanette wax   **1 dollop** Vitamin E

Waters:
    50 ml Geranium water
    300 ml Distilled water

Essential Oils:
    30 drops Eucalyptus   **20 drops** Rosemary
    30 drops Peppermint   **4 drops** Myrrh
    15 drops Black pepper

Preservative:
    1 dollop Grapefruit seed extract

METHOD:
Follow the *Basic Instructions*.

TO APPLY:
- Apply twice daily to the feet and calves for optimal results.

ADDING PLEASURE:
Every few weeks treat yourself to a reflexology treatment

Anti-Fungal Treatment

This topical treatment helps fight fungus on your toes and toenails. It does not cure toenail infection (the nail can be removed easily right down to the bed since the tissue is dead) but rather gets rid of the fungus on the skin, around the nails. To prevent further problems, avoid walking barefoot in public areas, such as locker rooms. In addition, keep your feet dry, wear cotton socks and change them frequently if your feet get wet.

INGREDIENTS

Foundational Ingredient:
   1 ml (20 drops) Vodka
Essential Oils:
   20 drops Myrrh
   4 ml Tea Tree

METHOD:
   1. Into a 5 ml dropper bottle, pour the vodka and myrrh.
   2. Fill the rest of the bottle with tea tree essential oil.

TO APPLY:
Use sparingly when needed between the toes and on the nails.

Natural Deodorant

Do you know that some of the most dangerous chemicals that we put on our body are in the form of antiperspirants? Yet daily, even our children are putting chemicals on their body and right in the area where the major lymphatic glands are to be found – no wonder there is so much breast cancer!

You even have to watch out for those rocks sold as "*aluminium-free* natural deodorant". You rub the rock under your arms. It works because the rock is made of magnesium-aluminium silicate!

Here is an alternative that will not just <u>act</u> as a natural deodorant, but will naturally detoxify the body, stimulate the immune system and also help the body to get rid of petro-chemicals that may already be stored in your organs.

Note: Those of you who have been using antiperspirants and deodorants for a long time may take some time to adjust, so please hang in there and let your body heal. Sometimes people sweat more than they used to (this should rectify in a short while) as the essential oils clean out the lymphatic system and allow the body to detoxify. So re-apply the deodorant as often as is necessary, making sure you wash regularly (you may need to carry a supply of the *Wipes* from the 'Holiday Care' section).

Wild Woman Deodorant

INGREDIENTS

Foundational Ingredients:
    90 ml Witch Hazel
    10 ml Vegetable glycerin
    1 tsp. Sea salt
Essential Oils:
    9 drops Lemon
    5 drops Grapefruit
    3 drops Geranium
    3 drops Mandarin
    2 drops Cypress
    2 drops Lavender
    1 drop Clove
    1 drop Coriander
    1 drop Oregano

METHOD:

1. Mix the Witch Hazel, Sea salt and Vegetable glycerin together.

2. Add the essential oils and mix together with the above.

3. Store in a dark glass bottle, preferably with an atomizer spray.

Note: Both clove and oregano essential oils have the ability to dissolve petro chemicals. This is particularly useful in this Wild Women's Deodorant which permits the use of both of these essential oils placed right on the lymphatic glands under the armpits, making this product a natural chemical detoxifying agent for the body.

Special Care

For those of you who suffer from migraines, menstrual cramps, hot flashes, or other discomfort, there are methods of managing your pain:

- Massage
- Exercise
- Spending time in the company of other women
- Use the products in this section

Headache and Sinus Lotion

INGREDIENTS

Foundational Ingredients:
    15 ml *Experimental Basic Lotion*
Essential Oils:
    6 drops Basil
    6 drops Peppermint
    6 drops Lavender
    6 drops Eucalyptus

METHOD:
Mix the drops into the white lotion.

TO APPLY:

- Apply a dollop to the temples and on the back of the neck when needed.

123

Hemp Moon Flow Balm

It's that time of the month again
And I am in so much pain
What will make me calm?
It's hemp moon flow balm

Here is some help for those who have pain. Clary sage has an emmenagogue effect (increases blood flow) and the geranium is a natural hormone balancer.

INGREDIENTS

Foundational Ingredients:
  ½ oz. (30 ml) Beeswax
  1 tsp. Shea Butter
  20 ml Hemp Oil
  70 ml Apricot Kernel Oil
  1 dollop Vitamin E
Essential Oils:
  20 drops Clary Sage
  20 drops Geranium

METHOD:
1. Melt the beeswax, shea butter and carrier oils in a double boiler. When it is almost melted, add the vitamin E, stirring all the time.

2. When the waxes and oils are completely melted, remove from the heat.

3. Add the essential oils and immediately pour into sterilized jars.

To Apply:

Apply liberally as often as needed to the abdomen and lower back.

Wild Yam Root Cream

Wild yam is a natural source of a progesterone precursor (diosgenin) that matches the composition of the body's progesterone to...

Balance Female Hormones!

Progesterone is helpful in:

- PMS and menstrual irregularity.

- Menopausal hot and cold flashes.

- Mood swings and depression.

- Balances skin moisture.

- Helps with stretch marks.

- Post-partum depression.

INGREDIENTS

Foundational Ingredients:
>**50 ml** *Experimental Basic Cream*
>**3.5 ml** Wild Yam Root Tincture

To Apply:

- Apply ¼ tsp. three times per day, to parts of the body where richer deposits of fatty tissue are found (like the buttocks, the upper arm or thigh).

- Rotate areas of application for better absorption (different places on different days or different times of the day).

- It's important to note your absorption time, as less than two minutes indicates a greater need. Therefore, apply more often (up to three times per day) if you notice cream disappearing in less than two minutes.

- Apply up to three times a day until your average absorption time increases to four minutes. Then reduce the number of applications.

PART
SEVEN

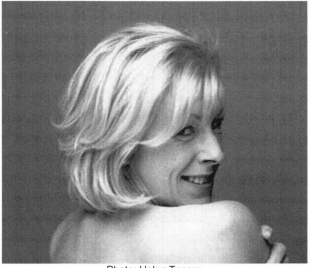

Photo: Helen Tansey

Hair Care

Taking care of your hair is important as we age because it is one of the ways we can signal that we are still young.

Here are some ways we can take extra care with our hair to keep it healthy:

Wetting your hair with fresh water before you swim in public swimming pools will keep it from soaking up too much chlorine. Be sure to rinse hair well after your swim with fresh water.

Help hair regain strength and vitality with an anti-aging shampoo that fights damaging free radicals, such as the *Chamomile Shampoo*.

To condition your hair, use the *Jojoba Conditioner* or treat your hair to a *Conditioning Pack*, especially if you're colouring your hair.

Prevent heat damage by allowing hair to air-dry as much as possible and turn down the heat on your blow-dryer.

After bathing and washing your hair, rinse in the coldest water possible. (Beneficial for both the skin and general health care).

Why make your own shampoo?

Well, one reason would be sodium laurel sulphate (SLS). Ninety percent of all commercial shampoo uses a detergent called sodium laurel sulphate and sodium laureth sulphate, which makes up to 50% of the shampoo. Potentially, SLS is perhaps the most harmful ingredient in personal-care products today. SLS is used in testing labs as the standard to irritate the skin. Industrial uses of SLS include garage floor cleaners, engine degreasers and car wash soaps to name just a few. Studies show its danger potential to be great when used in personal care products. One study indicates that SLS is systemic, and can penetrate and be retained in the eye, brain, heart and liver, with potentially harmful long-term effects. It could retard healing, cause cataracts in adults, and keep children's eyes from developing properly. I could write a whole book on chemicals alone. This is just one dangerous chemical out of many that we should avoid.

Others used in personal care products to watch out for are propylene glycol (antifreeze), phenylenediamine, formaldehyde, benzene, synthetic fragrance, and don't forget those artificial colours (FD&C or D&C numbers).

Another factor to be aware of is that there are no labelling laws in Canada. You do not have to put a list of ingredients on the label and if there is a list of ingredients, there is no guarantee that it is the complete list. The health store brands are often the worst offenders in this regard.

Anyway, moving right along, let's play.

Experimental Basic Shampoo

INGREDIENTS

Foundational Ingredients:
    100 ml Distilled water
    1 pinch Citric acid powder
    50 ml Cornacopa
    ¼ tsp. Xanthan gum
    1 dollop Vegetable glycerin
    1 dollop Wheat protein
Preservative
    1 dollop Grapefruit seed extract

METHOD:
1. Heat the water and Citric acid, sprinkle the Xanthan Gum onto the water and stir in.

2. When the Xanthan Gum has dissolved in the water (I often use a handheld blender to quicken the process), mix in the Wheat protein, the Vegetable glycerin and the Grapefruit seed extract.

3. Add the Cornacopa.

4. Enhance with goodies such as essential oils (for this recipe, use a total of 10 drops essential oil) and, Vitamin E.

5. Bottle and label.

Sparkle and Shine Shampoo

This is suitable for all hair types.

INGREDIENTS

Foundational Ingredients:
>**800 ml** Distilled water
>**100 ml** Rose water
>**½ tsp.** Citric Acid
>**2 dsp. (20 ml)** Xanthan Gum
>**3 tsp.** Vegetable glycerin
>**1 dsp.** Wheat protein
>**500 ml** Cornacopa

Goodies:
>**8 drops** Nettle extract
>**5 drops** Horsetail extract

Essential Oils:
>**20 drops** Lemon
>**15 drops** Lavender
>**15 drops** Rosemary
>**4 drops** Sandalwood

Preservative:
>**1 dollop** Grapefruit seed extract

METHOD:
Follow the instructions for the *Experimental Basic Shampoo* above.

Balancing Shampoo

This shampoo is for normal to oily hair.

INGREDIENTS

Foundational ingredients:
    800 ml Distilled water
    100 ml Orange blossom water
    ½ tsp. Citric acid
    2 dsp. (20 ml) Xanthan Gum
    3 tsp. Vegetable glycerin
    1 dsp. Seaweed extract
    500 ml Cornacopa
Goodies:
    5 drops Nettle extract
    5 drops Horsetail extract
    5 drops Coltsfoot extract
Essential Oils:
    24 drops Orange
    17 drops Rosemary
    4 drops Patchouli
Preservative:
    1 dollop Grapefruit seed extract

METHOD:
Follow the instructions given for the *Experimental Basic Shampoo* above.

Chamomile Shampoo

For normal to dry hair. This shampoo is especially helpful for those suffering from eczema or psoriasis.

INGREDIENTS

Foundational Ingredients:
   900 ml Distilled water
   100 ml Rose water
   ½ tsp. Citric Acid
   2 dsp. (20 ml) Xanthan Gum
   3 tsp. Vegetable glycerin
   1 dsp. Wheat protein
   500 ml Cornacopa
Goodies:
   8 drops Nettle extract
Essential Oils:
   40 drops Roman Chamomile
Preservative:
   1 dollop Grapefruit seed extract

METHOD:
Follow the instructions given for the *Experimental Basic Shampoo* above.

Conditioners

Hair that is dry, brittle tangles easily and is in need of nourishment might need some extra loving care. One natural way would be to rinse the hair with Cider vinegar (then again with clear water), but dry, damaged hair often needs extra help. For those with lank oily hair, just condition the ends if necessary. This conditioner also balances the Ph balance of the hair which will result in shiny, bouncy hair that is not weighed down.

Afterwards comb the hair starting at the lowest point of the tangled area one section of hair at a time.

Experimental Basic Conditioner

INGREDIENTS

Waxes and Oils:
> **1 tsp.** Conditioning wax emulsifier

Waters:
> **100 ml** Distilled water

Preservative:
> **1 dollop** Grapefruit seed extract

METHOD:
1. Heat up the water in a stainless steel saucepan.
2. Add the emulsifying wax to the hot water and heat until all the wax has melted.
3. Remove the pot from the heat source.
4. Stir until cool.
5. Add the Grapefruit seed extract, goodies and essential oils.
6. Bottle and label.

Jojoba Conditioner

Rich in ingredients which supply nutrients to the hair. Seaweed and Nettle extract help repair damaged hair. Jojoba oil coats the hair shaft to provide additional protection.

INGREDIENTS

Waxes and oils:
> **7 tsp.** Conditioning wax emulsifier

Waters:
> **800 ml** Distilled water
> **200 ml** Lemon balm water
> **½ tsp.** Citric acid
> **1 tsp.** Seaweed extract

Preservative:
> **1 dollop** Grapefruit seed extract

Goodies and Essential Oils:
> **½ tsp.** Jojoba Oil
> **1 dollop** Vitamin E
> **5 drops** Nettle extract
> **1 dollop** D-Panthenol (B5)
> *If the hair is blonde, add:*
> **20 drops** Roman chamomile
> *For graying or dark hair, add:*
> **20 drops** Rosemary

METHOD:
1. Heat the waters, Seaweed extract and Citric acid.
2. Add emulsifying wax to the hot water. Heat until melted.
3. Remove the pot from the heat source. Stir until cool.
4. Add the Grapefruit seed extract, Jojoba oil, Vitamin E, nutritive and essential oils.

Styling Gel

This is an alcohol-free gel that holds your hair in place. As an added bonus, it has amazing revitalizing and re-mineralizing properties for the scalp and hair. It is suitable for all hair types.

INGREDIENTS

Foundational Ingredient
> **100 ml** Seaweed gel

Essential Oils
> **10 drops** Rosemary
> **6 drops** Lemon
> **3 drops** Patchouli

METHOD:
Gently heat up the gel until it is melted and add the essential oils.

TO APPLY:
Apply a small amount (about the size of a coin) as you would any styling gel.

Note: Lemon essential oil bleaches the hair naturally especially in the sun. Omit it from the recipe if you do not wish to have this special effect.

> Note: A goodie is a nutrient (i.e., herbal extracts or carrier oils such as St. John's Wort or Calendula oil.)

Hair Treatments

Just like the skin, our hair reflects our inner health, so good nutrition is paramount in having glorious shiny tresses. We can also help our hair along with the application of conditioning packs. Salt water, chlorine, and the weather in general affect our hair, and, as we get older more and more women turn to colouring their hair to maintain their youthfulness. With all of these challenges, it is difficult to maintain the shine and bounce we once took for granted. Here are some treatments to help you keep your hair healthy.

Champagne Rinse

This makes a great finishing rinse to give your hair shine, making it glossy and healthy.

INGREDIENTS

> ½ **cup** Champagne (or sparkling wine such as the *Cremants* of Burgundy, the Spanish *Cava*s, or Italian *Spumantes*)
> ½ **cup** Stout beer (like *Black Velvet* or *Guinness*)

METHOD:
Mix the champagne and stout together.

TO APPLY:
Pour over your 'just shampooed' hair (do not use conditioner), rinse, dry and style as usual.

Clay Hair Pack

Natural clays that we use as masks on the skin, also function as deep conditioners for your hair. Clay cleanses the pores on your scalp which is beneficial for oily hair and also helps to prevent dandruff.

INGREDIENTS

2 dsp. Facial clay (such as *French green* or *Kaolin*)
1 tsp. Cider vinegar
1 tsp. Rose water

METHOD:
Mix the Rose water, clay and Cider vinegar together into a smooth paste.

TO APPLY:
Massage into your scalp and hair. Leave the mask on for 15 minutes, then rinse well with warm water, use no soap and dry gently.

Conditioning Packs

Any of the fruit facials (especially the *Banana, Avocado, Strawberries & Cream facials)* mentioned in part five, under masks and fruit facials can also be used as conditioning packs.

TO APPLY:
Simply rinse hair with warm water and massage the fruit facial mixture of your choice into hair and scalp. Cover hair with plastic wrap - a plastic bag or an old shower cap will do. Leave on for 15 minutes, then before rinsing, apply your shampoo to remove the conditioning pack, rinse and style your hair as usual.

For extra dry or damaged hair: Add 1 tablespoon of either sweet almond, sesame or melted coconut oils to one of the conditioning pack mixtures.

For oily hair: add 1 tsp. of lemon juice to one of the conditioning pack mixtures.

For other treatments, see *The Creamy Craft of Cosmetic Making* book.

Holiday Care

Whether you prefer the sun, sand or snow, taking care of your skin can be a challenge when you are on holiday. When travelling, it is especially important to maintain your beauty routine since even 'good' stress can impact the skin. To minimize the amount of products you need to carry, our *Ultra-Firming Gel* can be used as a three-in-one formula for day, night and eye-treatment as it helps simplify life.

Be aware that sunscreens are one of the most dangerous things you can put on your skin, but more about that later.

Survival in the Woods

"No See 'Em" Bug Spray

This bug spray is all-natural and allows you protection from pesky insects as well as harmful pesticides.

INGREDIENTS

Foundational Ingredients:
>   **5 ml** Cider vinegar
>   **5 ml** Witch Hazel
>   **100 ml** Distilled water

Essential Oils:
>   **8 drops** Citronella
>   **4 drops** Thyme
>   **4 drops** Lavender
>   **4 drops** Pine
>   **4 drops** Peppermint
>   **3 drops** Cedarwood

METHOD:

1. Mix the essential oils into the Cider vinegar and Witch Hazel, shake gently.

2. Add the water.

3. Store in a glass bottle.

TO APPLY:

* Shake before using and spray on exposed areas of the skin – especially arms and legs. Don't forget to spray the tender areas around the ankles and feet.

Baby Bug Spray

This bug spray helps you to protect little ones.

INGREDIENTS

Foundational Ingredients:
> **5 ml** Cider vinegar
> **5 ml** Witch Hazel
> **40 ml** Lavender water

Essential Oils:
> **3 drops** Roman Chamomile
> **3 drops** Lemongrass
> **3 drops** Mandarin
> **1 drop** Lavender

METHOD:
1. Mix the essential oils into the Cider vinegar and Witch Hazel, shake gently.

2. Add the water and store in a glass bottle.

TO APPLY:
* Shake before using and spray on skin.

Boo Boo Soother

This ointment is a wonderful healer for any cuts, sores, rashes and even eczema and psoriasis. It is even gentle enough for babies. Good for anything under a band-aid.

INGREDIENTS

Foundational Ingredients:
    ½ **oz.** Beeswax
    5ml (1 tsp.) Shea butter
    60 ml Apricot Kernel Oil
    20 ml Calendula infused oil
    10 ml St. John's Wort oil
    1 dollop Vitamin E
Essential Oils:
    5 drops Tea tree
    5 drops Lavender
    2 drops Myrrh

METHOD:
1. Melt the beeswax, shea butter and carrier oils in a double boiler. When it is almost melted, add the Vitamin E, stirring all the time.

2. When the waxes and oils are completely melted, remove from the heat.

3. Add the essential oils.

4. Immediately pour into sterilized jars.

Wipes

Keeping clean can be hard whilst in the woods.
Yet, once again this book has the goods.

Once a year, I go off into the woods to do ceremony which often means that I am away from a shower or bath and therefore going without washing for a few days. Yet people often comment that I look clean and smell good afterwards. Here's how I do it!

These wipes are not just useful for the woods but handy whenever travelling. They also make great baby wipes.

INGREDIENTS

> *Rose Geranium Freshener*
> Paper Towels

METHOD:
Cut the paper towels into quarters. Fold each piece in quarters again, soak in the freshener. Store in a plastic zip lock bag.

Body Freshener

Another way of cleaning oneself is to travel with a bottle of *Rose Geranium Freshener* and cotton pads. Simply use them to freshen and clean the body as need. Afterwards spray on the Wild Woman's Deodorant.

Tip: If you happen to get a mosquito or black fly bite, an immediate anti-itch relief is to apply rose geranium essential oil neat (directly) to the area.

Jet Lag Serum

To jump start your get up and go.

INGREDIENTS

Foundational Ingredients:
    7.5 ml Seaweed extract
Essential Oils:
    5 drops Lavender
    4 drops Geranium
    4 drops Grapefruit
    3 drops Lemon

METHOD:
Add the essential oils to the Seaweed extract.

TO APPLY:
This can be used in a couple of different ways:

- Applied as a moisturiser to the skin on the face and neck.
- For a revitalizing bath, add 5 ml of the serum to the bath water and soak for at least 10 minutes.

Survival in the Sun

The most obvious way to avoid telltale signs of aging is to stay inside. But just as important to health is the need to absorb the sun's rays to get sufficient vitamin D and to perk up moods, which often means lingering in its warmth and enjoying the glow for far longer than may be wise.

While overdoing it can ruin your skin, exposure to the sun for at least 30 minutes a day is necessary. As we age, the ability of the skin to convert vitamin D to its active form decreases. Vitamin D3, a pro-hormone, is important in the absorption of calcium and other vitamins. (best produced by sunlight on the skin) and recent research has shown that many people are lacking this important vitamin.

By taking a sun-bath (in your bathing suit in the summer), your skin will work with the sun to produce 10,000 IU in one hour. In the fall, winter and spring, all Canadians and Northern Europeans should boost their intake of vitamin D with-supplements.

Interestingly, supplements of vitamin D3 of 2,000 IU's taken with breakfast has been found to help protect against sunburn. Fascinatingly, eating cooked tomatoes with your breakfast also provides a natural sunscreen!

If you plan to spend time in the sun, it is important that you find a sunscreen that is compatible with your skin. Many people are allergic to specific sunscreen components yet they are perfectly fine with others.

Some people prefer to use physical sunscreens as opposed to more chemical options. Physical sunscreens may be preferable to chemical options because they do not interact with the cells. Physical sunscreens are made of tiny little zinc or titanium particles that act like tiny mirrors to reflect the sun's rays.

In contrast, chemical sunscreens work by interacting with the skin cells and absorbing the sun's rays. Some say that many chemical sunscreens increase cancer by generating free radicals. Others may create strong hormone reactions, and be responsible for serious sexual dysfunctions as well as cancer.

Many chemical sunscreens do not block UVA radiation, which increases the rate of melanoma (a kind of skin cancer), but not sunburn. Additionally, sunscreens block UVB, and, if used consistently, can cause a deficiency of vitamin D.

Chemical sunscreens include:

Benzophenones Compounds that absorb ultraviolet light that are often used in inks, imaging, and coatings in the print industry. They also prevent light from penetrating the plastic on products such as perfumes and soaps. May be carcinogenic (for example, oxybenzone, is a suspected carcinogen).

Cinnamates People with sensitivities to balsam of Peru, tolu balsam, coca leaves, cinnamic aldehyde, and cinnamic oil can also be sensitive to the cinnamates.

Salicylates Protects only against a small part of the UVB spectrum so it has to be used in

Menthyl anthranilate high concentrations. Used in the production of dyes, pigments and saccharin. Its esters are used in corrosion inhibitors for metals and mold inhibitors in soya sauce.

Avobenzone. Degrades significantly in light, resulting in less protection over time. The UVA light in a day of sunlight in a temperate climate is sufficient to break down most of the compound (e.g. following one hour of exposure to sunlight).

The harmful chemicals that go into protective UV creams are a serious concern.

In 1997, Europe, Canada and Australia banned most sunscreens except these three: avobenzone, titanium dioxide and zinc oxide. Others may still be in use in the U.S. where many holiday-goers travel for their sun vacations.

Adding to the problem is that when people use chemical sunscreens daily, large amounts of these chemicals enter the bloodstream through the skin.

A natural full spectrum sun block such as titanium dioxide or zinc oxide (yes, the white stuff surfer's use) will block out UVA and UVB rays by acting as a physical barrier. They are less irritating and longer lasting.

What about a Suntan?

While some people practically worship their tanning-bed (and it shows in their skin's texture), you also need to be wary of self-tanners and their chemicals. Self-tanners work by increasing the-pigment in the skin.

So, be wise and take care of your skin.

Recovery from Sun Damage

Most of us have some sun damage. Whether its freckles, age spots or wrinkles, you've got photo-aging, or premature aging this damage is caused by over exposure to the sun.

However, note that the skin has an incredible ability to repair itself. In fact, studies have shown impressive improvements in sun-damaged skin after only two years of sun avoidance.

To speed the repair process along, eat an acid/alkaline balanced diet, and take antioxidant and anti-inflammatory supplements such as vitamins C, E, and coenzyme Q-10. Using lotions containing essential oils such as carrot seed, frankincense, lemon/lime or mandarin, and using powerful antioxidants such as vitamin E, and vitamin C ester, is also highly recommended.

Get Ready for Summer

1. Exfoliate your skin

2. Banish spider veins and brown spots by visiting an electrologist

3. Prevent and help reverse sun damage by using the *Sun Cream* or the *Sun Oil.*

4. Remove unwanted hair

5. Remove stubborn fat deposits with a lymphatic drainage massage

6. Exercise and maintain a healthy diet

Sun Cream

This is a double action cream that can be used both before and after sunbathing. As well as protecting the skin, it soothes and heals at the same time.

INGREDIENTS

Waxes and Oils:
> **1 oz.** Lanette Wax
> **1 tsp.** Shea Butter
> **10 ml** Coconut Oil
> **60 ml** Sesame Oil
> **1 dollop** Carrot Root Oil
> **1 dollop** Vitamin E

Waters:
> **700 ml** Distilled water
> **50 ml** Aloe Vera

Essential Oils:
> **4 drops** Lavender
> **2 drops** Roman Chamomile

METHOD:
Follow the *Basic Instructions.*

TO APPLY:
Apply as often as needed wherever you need protection from the sun.

Note: For even more protection, add 1 tsp. of zinc oxide powder to the above cream and mix well.

Sun Oil

Some people prefer to use a sun product that makes their skin glisten in the sunlight. Sesame oil has an SPF of 4. This oil can be used both before and after sunbathing. As well as protecting the skin, it soothes and heals at the same time.

INGREDIENTS

40 ml Sesame Oil
1 dollop Carrot Root Oil
1 dollop Vitamin E

Essential Oils (*Optional*):
10 drops of your choice of any essential oil except citrus oils (as they are photo toxic).

METHOD:
Simply combine the oils.

TO APPLY:
Apply as often as needed wherever you need protection from the sun.

Sunburn Remedy

To ease the pain of sunburn, try these natural remedies:

- Mash strawberries or cucumber, pat on and leave for ½ hour.

- Mix equal parts of baking soda and water, pat on and leave for ½ hour.

- Mix ¼ cup of yogurt with 2 tbsp. Rose water and splash over the skin.

- Pull a leaf/stem of the Aloe Vera plant off, cut the stem at a wide point, and squeeze out the contents. Apply the resulting gel directly to the skin.

PART NINE

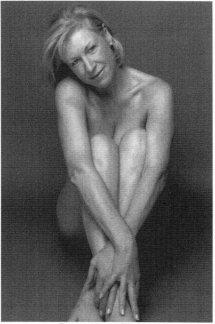

Photo: Helen Tansey

Es-sensual Sexuality

For optimum beauty and health, how one feels about oneself shows up in his/her sexual vibrancy.

Essential oils though, do have an effect on one's libido. Here are some true life stories just to make a point.

Attraction Oils

At one of my workshops I was talking about one of my favourite essential oils Ylang ylang, (often called the cheap man's Jasmine), and how it was an aphrodisiac. So a student decided to douse himself in the oil. What happened? Well let's just say he had an interesting evening...

If you want to attract, and feel in the mood for love, use Ylang ylang extra (flower of flowers).

Other aphrodisiac oils include: Jasmine, Patchouli, Geranium, Rose, Clary sage and Sandalwood.

Apply 1 to 2 drops, (remember, they are very strong) as you would a fine perfume, on the pulse points. For example, dab a drop behind the ears, back of the knee, and the inside of the elbow.

How you feel about yourself definitely affects your magnetic attracting personality (MAP). So taking care of yourself is a must if you are to give off the right vibes, an aphrodisiac in itself.

Lover's Ceremony

Here is a lover's ceremony that I have put together for you to enjoy.

One way of getting in the mood for love is through the giving and receiving of massage. However, the massage does not always have to be given as a prelude to making love; it can be performed as a loving act just by itself. If you are celibate and/or do not have a partner, then celebrate and love your body by performing massage on yourself.

For the Lovers Ceremony, start with a tea ceremony, then shower or bathe together. Now each of you take turns massaging each other, taking your time.
Massaging can be hungry work so do be sure to allow the time to eat.

Make sure you prepare first. Create the massage oil you will be using ahead of time (see the blends below).

Before you start, create a special space with soft cushions, lighted candles, music and food to nibble on. The room should be warm and what could be better than to accent the room with a log fire. Make sure that you have some soft towels to cover the areas that you are not working on because unless it is sweltering hot, it is very easy for your lover to become chilled.

Beyond the massage oil, ingredients needed are, green tea and jasmine for the tea ceremony, and for the last part of the ceremony: whipped cream, slices of kiwi, orange and bananas, plus some strawberries.

1. TEA CEREMONY

Prepare the tea by putting 1 tsp. green tea and 1 drop of jasmine into a teapot. Now add 3-4 cups of boiling water to the tea leaves.

Sit opposite each other, drink a cup of the tea and let go of any stress and any thoughts that will take away from the pleasure to come.

2. BATHE OR SHOWER TOGETHER

Shower or bathe together with the luxurious *Afternoon Delight Body Wash.*

3. MASSAGE

One of the ways to use essential oils is through massage. We are sensuous beings and our bodies respond to being touched. It is important when giving the massage to be as comfortable as possible, so make sure that you have a cushion to kneel on.

Starting on your partners back, kneel at your lover's side and make sure that your hands are warm (you can rub them together to increase friction and warm them up). Slowly, pour some of the oil blend into the palm of your hand (approximately the size of a quarter or pound coin) and then rub your hands together. Now place your hands on either side of the spine on the lower back and spread the oil evenly over the back. With the palms flat and fingers pointing towards the head, slide them smoothly and firmly up the back to the neck then move your hands outwards to the point of the shoulders and lightly down the side of the back. Repeat many times. Now do TV massage, so named because this is usually what is shown on television when massage is performed. Place thumbs on either side of the spine and slowly work your way up the back circling with your thumb pads up and out, noting any tense spots (usually there are quite a few in the upper back). Be sure to stick to muscle groups and fleshy areas. Now let your imagination flow and don't just massage with your hands. Use your hair, and women your breasts. With your mouth, gently lick and nibble. When you have finished on the back, move on to the buttocks and the back of the legs.

Now turn your lover over and massage the front of the body in the same manner. Touch every part of the body, the feet, back of the knee, the ears and find pleasure spots that you never knew existed.

When you have finished, switch places and receive.

Now for the feast.

4. LICK THE PLATE CLEAN

We have already discovered how fruits rejuvenate the skin on the face. So here is an exotic way to use them on the body.

Start by applying 1 large dollop (1 dsp.) of the whipped cream on the following four chakras (the major energy centres in the body):

- The heart chakra which is at the tip of the sternum (just under the heart and in the centre):
- the solar plexus chakra which is at the navel;
- the *hara*, which is just above the pubic hairline, and finally
- on the first chakra. For men this is at the base of the penis (where it meets the body) and, on women the clitoris (where the genitals begin).

Now place pieces of fruit on each mound of whipped cream:

- at the heart place the kiwi fruit,
- on the navel place the sliced banana,
- on the hara place the orange and
- on the first chakra place a strawberry.

These colours reflect the colours in the aura of the chakras.

Now lick the plate clean.

Massage Oil

If giving an erotic massage or if pleasuring yourself, the essential oil of sandalwood blended in jojoba is sensuous, pleasurable and will not irritate sensitive areas.

Choose one of the blends below.

INGREDIENTS

Foundational ingredients
 30m1 infused vanilla bean oil or jojoba oil
 (for the erotic massage oil) 10 ml jojoba oil only

Essential Oils

SACRED SEX	SELF LOVE
3 drops Geranium	**2 drops** Rose
2 drops Patchouli	**1 drop** Sandalwood
3 drops Orange	**3 drops** Lavender
TANTRIC TEASER	VELVET PLEASURE
4 drops Jasmine	**4 drops** Ylang ylang
2 drops Bergamot	**2 drops** Bergamot
2 drops Clary sage	**6 drops** Sandalwood

EROTIC MASSAGE OIL

5 drops sandalwood

METHOD:
For all except the erotic massage oil, combine the essential oils with the 30 ml infused vanilla bean oil or

jojoba oil. For the erotic massage oil, combine the essential oil of sandalwood with 10 ml jojoba oil.

Anti-Aphrodisiac

Relaxes the body parts that other oils can't reach

A therapist friend of mine started to notice that he wasn't interested in sex anymore. He put it down to his age, 42 years old, perhaps he was past it? Well, one day whilst reading about marjoram essential oil he discovered that marjoram was an anti aphrodisiac. Now marjoram is an incredible pain reliever and my friend was using rather a lot of it in his massage treatments. Once he started using an alternative essential oil, he discovered that everything was back to status quo.

So, if you are in a position of enforced celibacy, or in need of a pain reliever, just put a couple of drops of marjoram essential oil in your bath and in your moisturiser and body lotions.

Appendix 1

Your notes and recipes

Your notes and recipes

Your notes and recipes

If you enjoyed this book, check out other books by the author.

The Creamy Craft of Cosmetic Making *with essential oils and their friends,* **2011** as well as being another cream making book, studies the use of essential oils and carrier oils in skin, body and hair care products. Also included is treatments for body care especially cellulite and fat reduction, along with a diet and plan of action. Care of the skin is covered including treatments for stretch marks, varicose veins and aches and pains.

The little Book of lipsticks, 2010 is a fun but practical book, which contains easy to follow recipes to make safe, all natural, professional quality lipsticks.
Included is the history and trivia of lipsticks, knowledge of the natural ingredients used, and how to apply the perfect lipstick.
Recipes included are: Baby pink, Cinnamon girl, Smitten and Chocolate kisses *(made with real chocolate).*

Coming soon: The Art of Soap Making, 2011 and The Art of Making Natural Makeup, 2012

Appendix 2
Bibliography

Bateman, Robert (2009) Bringing Nature Home *Vista Magazine*, Issue 65, p. 26-27.

Benham, Jan (1996) **The Creamy Craft of Cosmetic Making with essential oils and their friends** Toronto: The Aromashoppe.

Fackelmann, Kathleen. (2005) Stress can ravage the body, unless the mind says no: A positive outlook can reduce impact of stress on health. *USA Today*, March 22, 2005. http://www.usatoday.com/educate/college/firstyear/articles/20050327.htm

Ganora, Lisa, (2004) The colors of vitality: antioxidants and phytonutrients in foods and herbs *New Life Journal*, June-July, 2004.

Meister, Mark, Chamberlain, Kristen, and Brown, Amanda (2006) Rejuvenating Nature in Commercial Culture and the Implications of the Green Commodity Form. In Depoe, Stephen P. (ed.) **The Environmental Communication Yearbook**. New Jersey: Lawrence Erlbaum, Chapter 5, pp. 91-106.

Perricone, Nicholas (2000) **The Wrinkle Cure: Unlock the Power of Cosmeceuticals for Supple, Youthful Skin.** Emmaus, PA: Rodale Books.

Regehr Clark, Hulda (1993) **The Cure for all Diseases**. San Diego, CA: ProMotion Publishing.

Talbot, Margaret (2009) Nightmare Scenario – Can We Learn to Rewrite Our Bad Dreams? *The New Yorker*, November 16, 2009, pp. 43-51.

Tolle, E. (2006) **A New Earth: Awakening to Your Life's Purpose**. London: Plume.

Appendix 3
Further Reading

Allen, David (2001) **Getting Things Done: The Art of Stress-Free Productivity** New York: Penguin

Baker, Dan (2003) **What Happy People Know: How the New Science of Happiness Can Change Your Life for the Better.** New York: St. Martin's Press.

Baker, Nena (2008) **The Body Toxic: How the Hazardous Chemistry of Everyday Things Threatens Our Health and Well-being** New York: North Point Press.

Balch, Phyllis A. (2006) **Prescription for Nutritional Healing**, Fourth Edition, New York: Avery.

Begoun, Paula (1994) **Don't Go to the Cosmetics Counter Without Me: An Eye Opening Guide to Brand Name Cosmetics.** Seattle: Beginning Press.

Canfield, Jack (1995) **The Aladdin Factor** New York: Berkley Publishing.

Covey, Stephen R. (2004) **The 7 Habits of Highly Effective People** New York: Free Press.

Covey, Stephen R., Roger Merrill, and Rebecca R. Merrill, (1994) **First Things First: To Live, to Love, to Learn, to Leave a Legacy.** New York: Simon and Schuster

Diamond, Denise (1982) **The Complete Book of Flowers** California: North Atlantic books.

Frankl, Viktor E. (2004) **Man's Search for Meaning.** London: Random House / Rider.

Hewitt, Fran and Hewitt, Les (2003) **The Power of Focus for Women.** Deerfield Beach, FL: Health Communications.

Lyons, James R. (2009) **The Brown Fat Revolution: Trigger Your Body's Good Fat To Lose Weight And Be Healthier**. London: St. Martin's Press.

Malkan, Stacy (2007) **Not Just a Pretty Face: The Ugly Side of the Cosmetic Industry.** Gabriola Island, BC: New Society

Mate, Gabor (2003) **When the Body Says No: The Cost of Hidden Stress.** Toronto: Knopf Canada.

Millman, Dan J. **(2000) Way of the Peaceful Warrior** Novato, CA: H.J. Kramer.

Millman, Dan J. (1999) **Body Mind Mastery: Training for Sport and Life.** Novato, CA: New World Library.

Nisker, Andrew (dir.) (2009) *Chemerical.* Toronto: Take Action Films.

Schapiro, Mark (2007) **Exposed: The Toxic Chemistry of Everyday Products and What's at Stake for American Power.** White River Junction, VT: Chelsea Green Publishing.

Seligman, Martin P. (2002) **Authentic Happiness: Using the New Positive Psychology to Realize Your Potential for Lasting Fulfillment**. New York: Free Press.

Sharma, Robin (2006) **The Greatness Guide: 101 Lessons for Making What's Good at Work and in Life Even Better.** New York: Harper Collins Publishers.

Smith, Rick and Lourie, Bruce (2009) **Slow Death by Rubber Duck: The Secret Danger of Everyday Things**. Toronto: Knopf Canada.

Tolle, Eckhart (2005) **The Power of Now: A Guide to Spiritual Enlightenment.** New York: New World Library.

Wildwood, Chrissie, (1994) **Sensual Aromatherapy: Essential oils for lovers**. London: Headline.

Winter, Ruth M. (2009) **Consumers Dictionary of Cosmetic Ingredients**. New York: Crown Publishing.

Appendix 4
We offer Holistic Health Practitioner Diploma and Aroma Cosmetology courses.

We also carry supplies for making your own line of cosmetics and custom make for companies around the world.

**Organic Skin, Hair, Body Care Products
Makeup – natural lipsticks and mineral makeup
Natural cold pressed Soap**
Canada
The Aroma shoppe Ltd.,
2092 Queen St. E.,
Toronto, Ontario
M4E 1E1
Tel: (416) 698 5850
E-mail: janbenham@gmail.com
www.aromashoppe.com

Great Britain
18 Milton Crescent,
Ravenshead, Notts.
NGI5 9BA
Tel: 01623 797100
E-mail: janbenham@gmail.com

Members of the International Federation of Professional Aromatherapists, UK, The International Federation of Holistic Therapists, UK, and the Canadian Examining Board of Health Care Practitioners, Canada.

Appendix 5
Index of recipes

...Cont'd next page